Tuberculosis
voices of the unheard

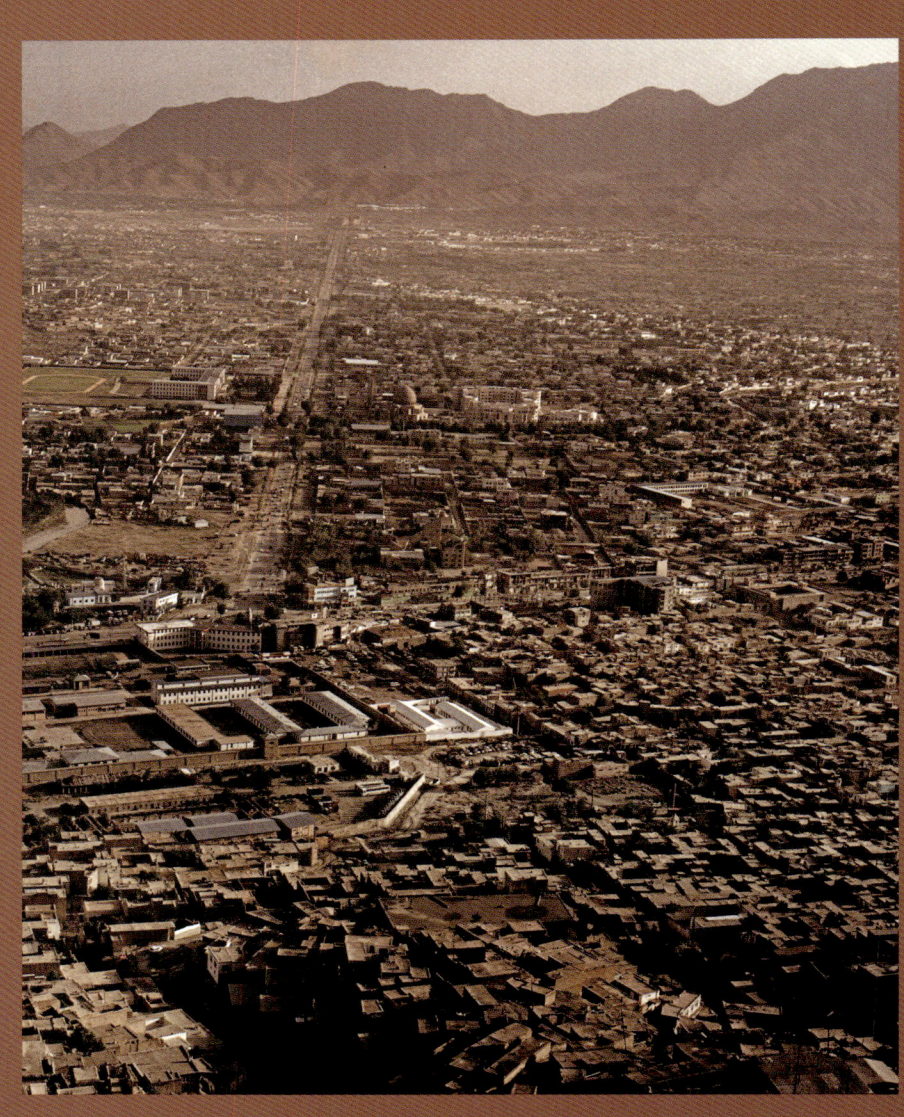

In the Name of God, the Compassionate, the Merciful

Foreword

As public health experts, we use numbers to present the tremendous size of the tuberculosis dilemma: 2 million deaths in the world every year and 120 000 deaths in the WHO Eastern Mediterranean Region alone. These are, without doubt, extremely important and disturbing statistics that describe the enormity of the challenge we confront. However, away from numerical depiction of the problem, its human face needs to be recognized and emphasized. The suffering caused by tuberculosis has many aspects, social and economic. It is imperative that we understand the suffering and hardship tuberculosis imposes on the people who have the disease and on their families, and the struggle each faces to cope with the arduous changes in their lives as a result.

This pictorial book, *Tuberculosis: voices of the unheard* presents that human face of tuberculosis. Indeed, each face clearly communicates the measure of suffering in each person living with tuberculosis. They are from Afghanistan; women and men, young and old––each is a victim of tuberculosis, a disease we have known for centuries and a disease that is completely preventable and curable. Some of these people, unfortunately, are among the many dying every day around the world. The Government of Afghanistan and the World Health Organization are responding to this challenge, supported by international tuberculosis advocates like Anna Cataldi, Ambassador of the Stop TB Partnership and a former United Nations Messenger of Peace and Ricardo Venturi, a renowned photographer. They visited Afghanistan in June 2007 not just to bring these images of the misery wrought by a preventable disease but to give a voice to those who cannot make themselves heard.

Women are at the centre of this agony. In Afghanistan, 70% of tuberculosis patients are female. They are mothers, daughters, wives and children. Their pain deepens when their fathers, husbands and siblings suffer from the same affliction. Ricardo Venturi's photographs not only detail the life of ordinary Afghan women affected by tuberculosis but also portray the vulnerability and neglect haunting their lives. The photographs, at the same time, take the viewer on a journey of discovery of the meaning of suffering in conflict-ravaged countries, so expressively described by Anna Cataldi in her powerful story, in the opening pages.

Each face among the photographs vividly asks us to think of what can be done to alleviate the pain. Tuberculosis is indeed totally preventable and curable, and thus these faces should be wearing smiles and radiating life. In fact, these photographs compel us to consider that this is the time to act, to stop the loss and contribute towards halting tuberculosis. I hope you too can hear the unheard voices in the photographs and will respond to their call.

Hussein A. Gezairy MD FRCS
Regional Director for the Eastern Mediterranean

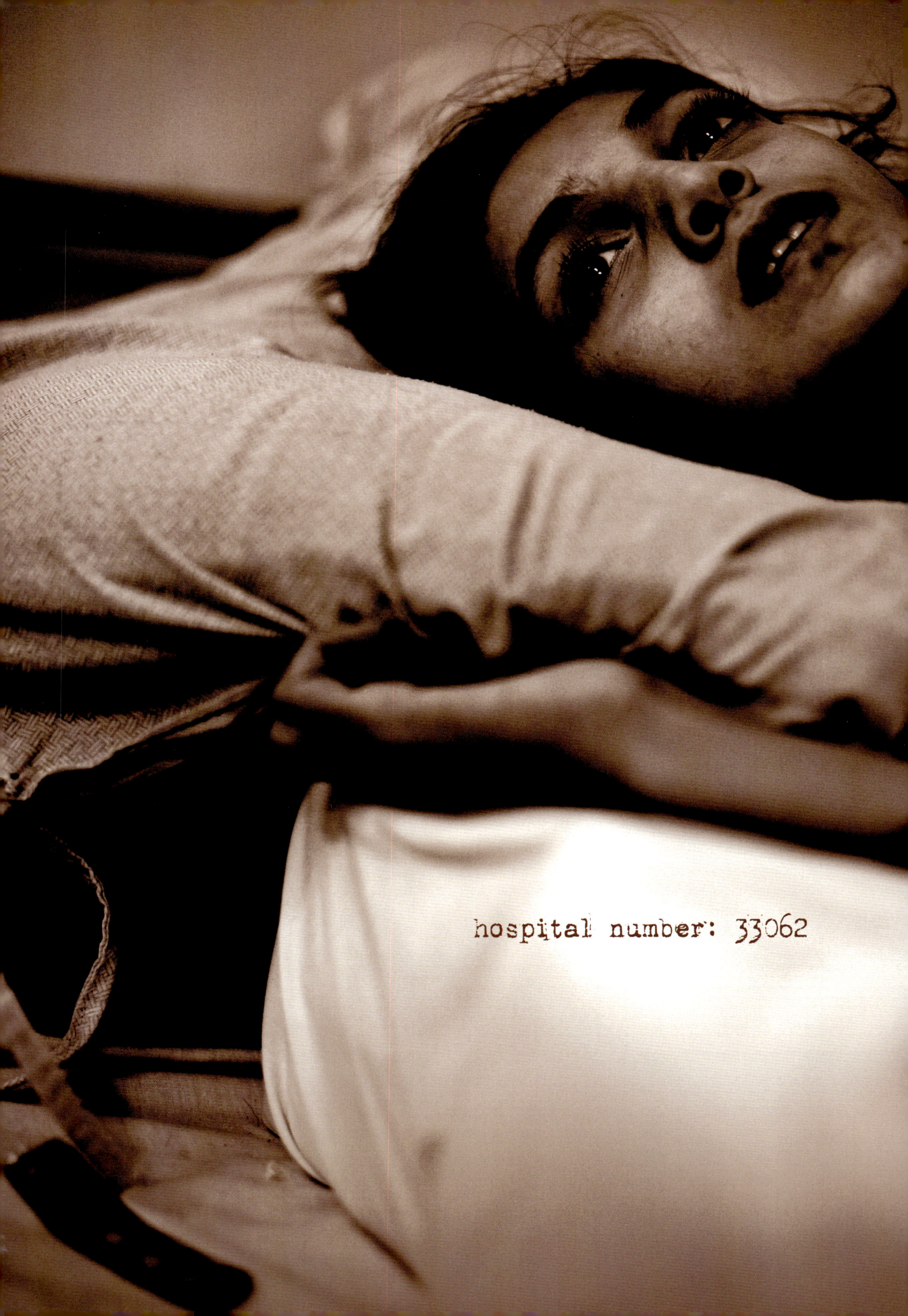

Fazilla arrived at the hospital on May 19, 2007
After two years of false opinions, she was finally
diagnosed with tubercular spondylitis

She is not the only one...
Every year tuberculosis kills 15,000 people in
Afghanistan alone, nearly 13,000 are women
who endure the worst living conditions

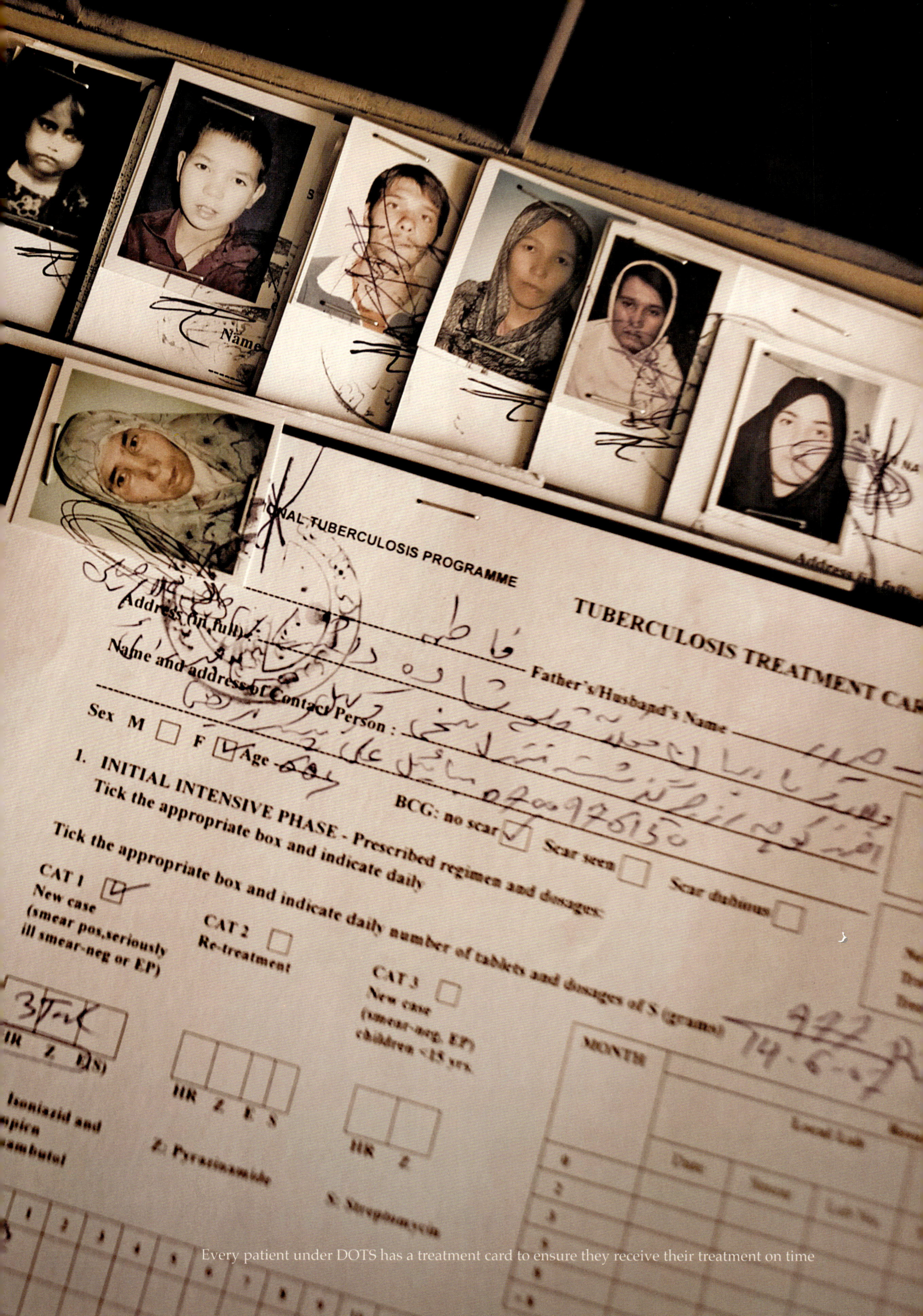

Every patient under DOTS has a treatment card to ensure they receive their treatment on time

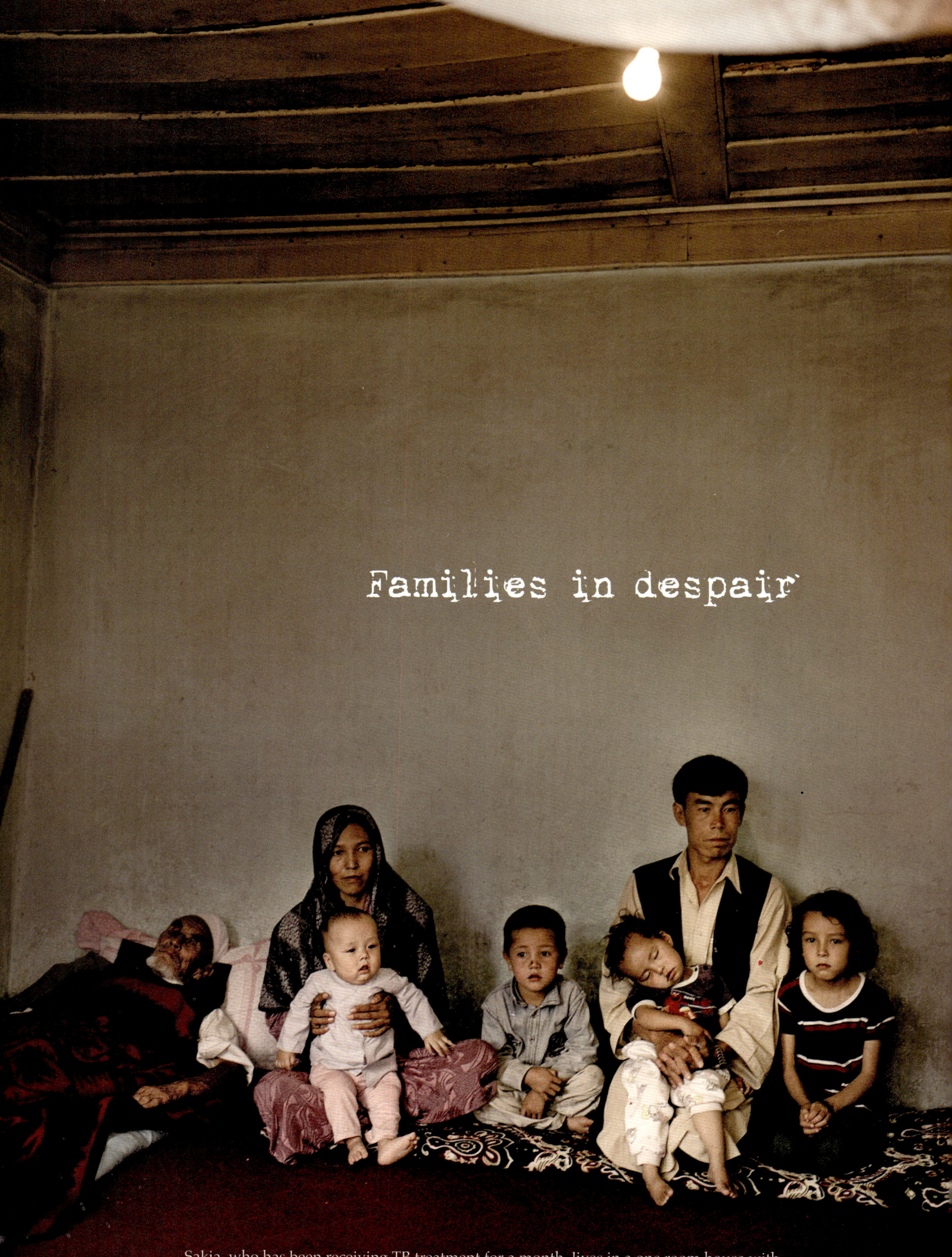

Families in despair

Sakia, who has been receiving TB treatment for a month, lives in a one room house with her grandfather, who is blind, and seven others; her mother died of TB 10 years ago

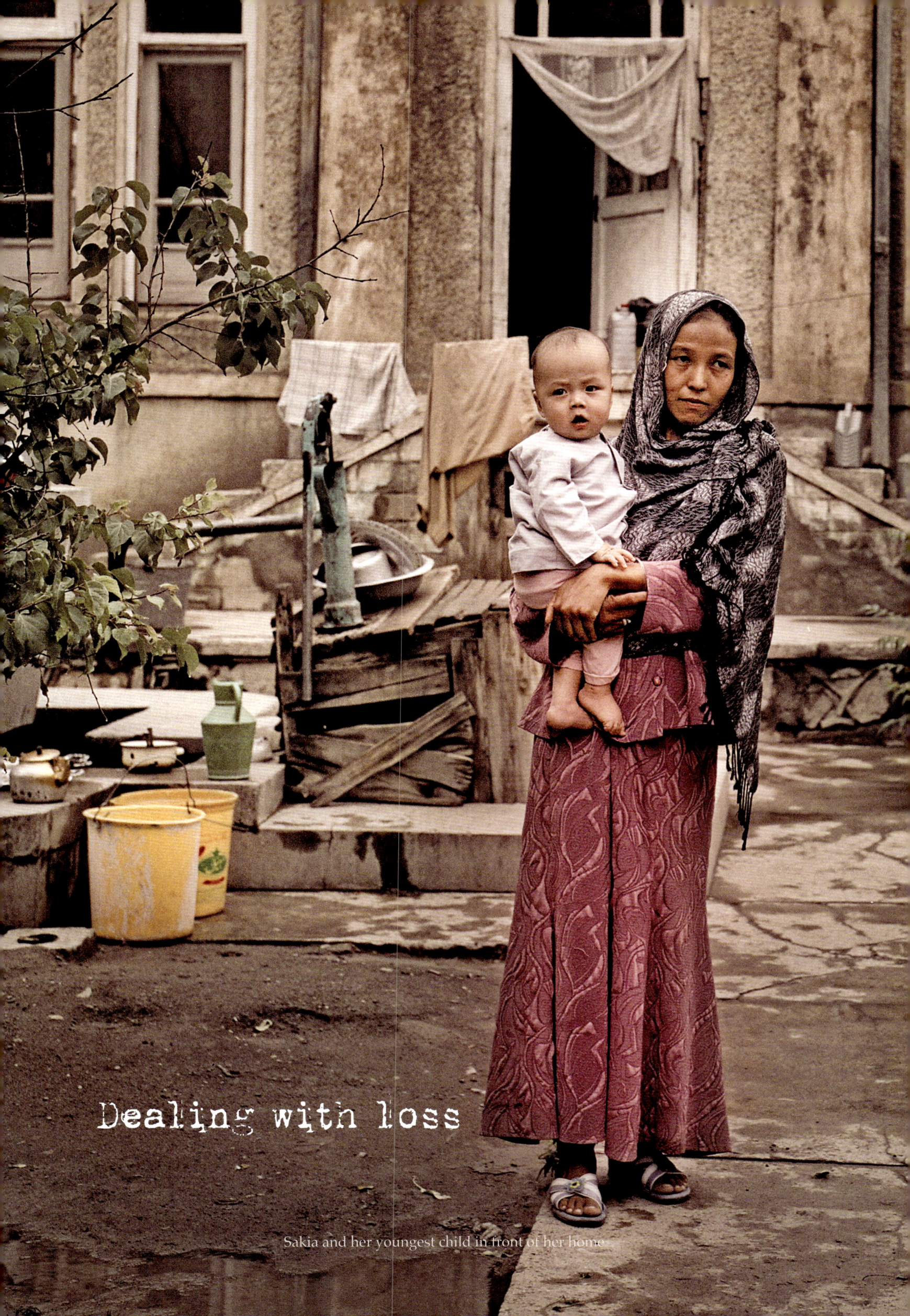

Dealing with loss

Sakia and her youngest child in front of her home.

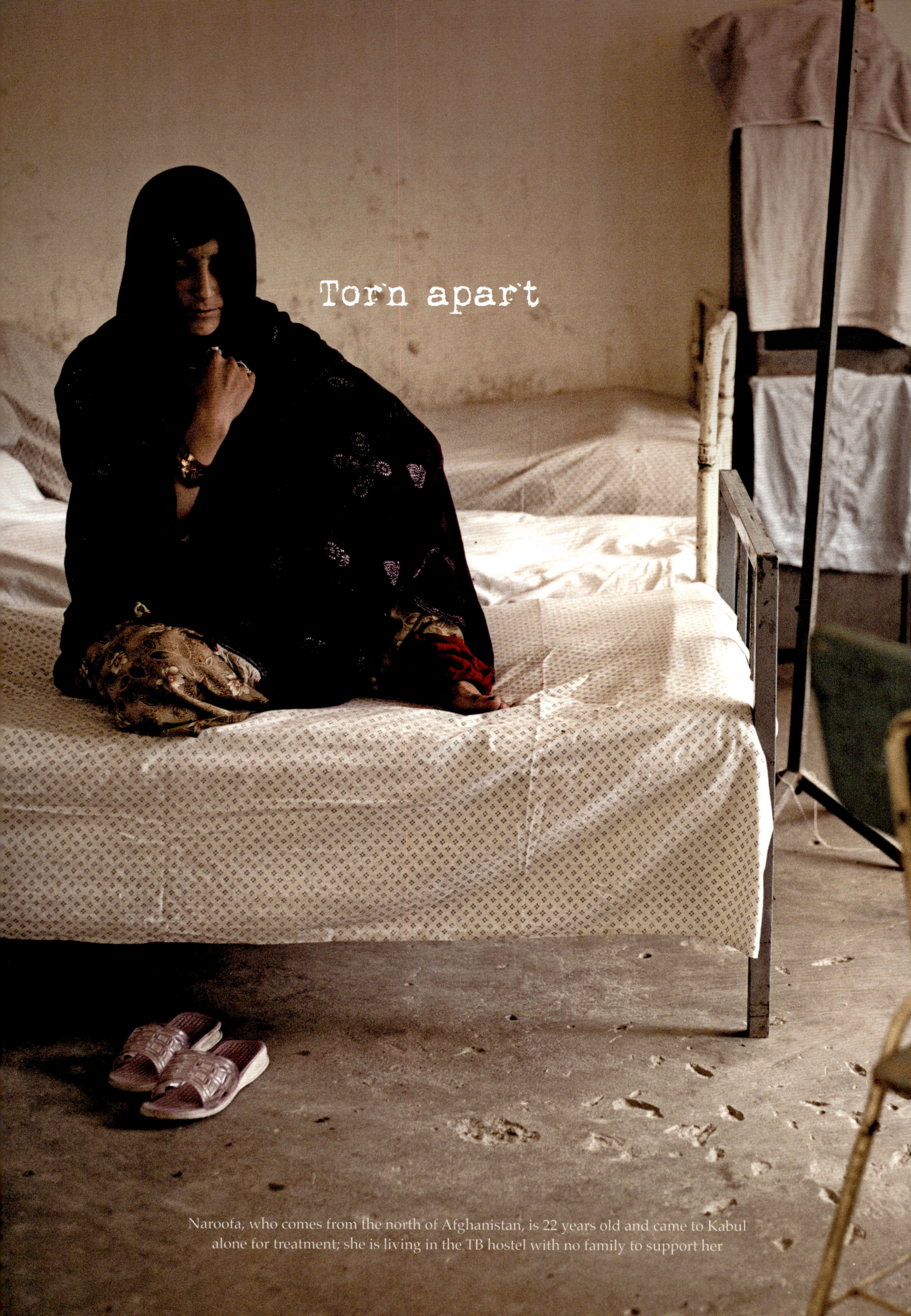

Torn apart

Naroofa, who comes from the north of Afghanistan, is 22 years old and came to Kabul alone for treatment; she is living in the TB hostel with no family to support her

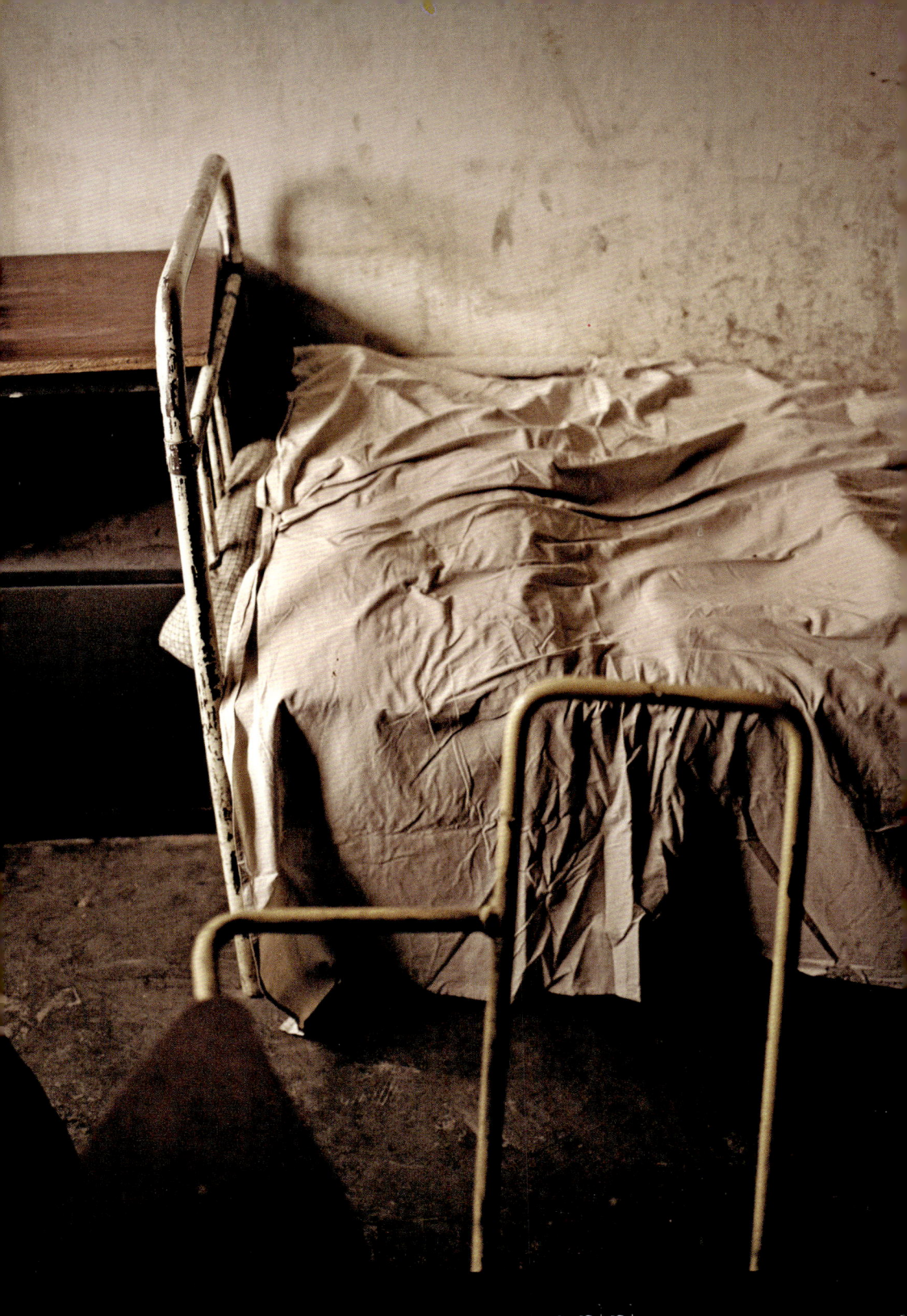

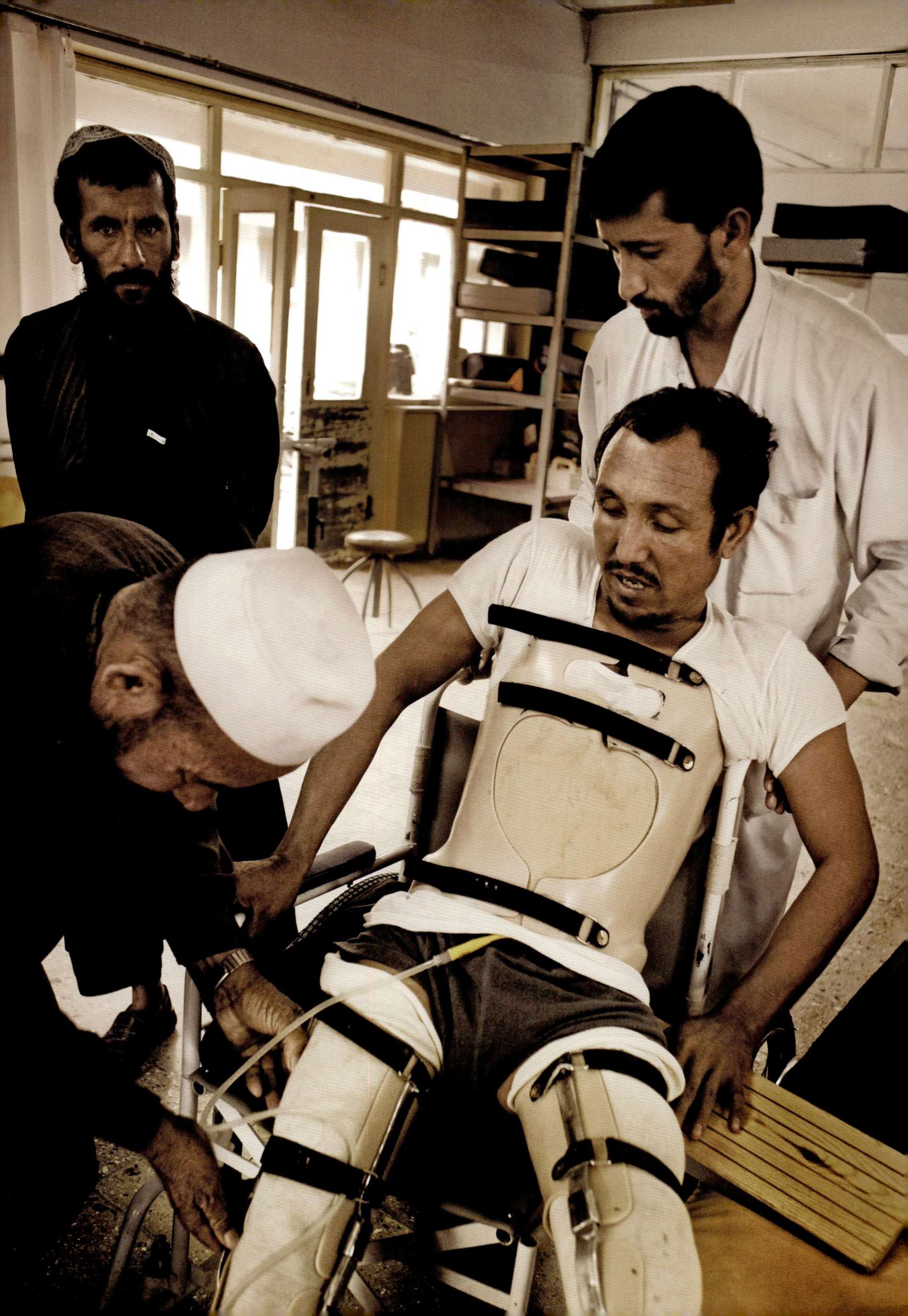

...or a new beginning...

if we act now

Omar has spinal TB and is paralysed but doctors are hopeful
he will recover 70% of his mobility with rehabilitation

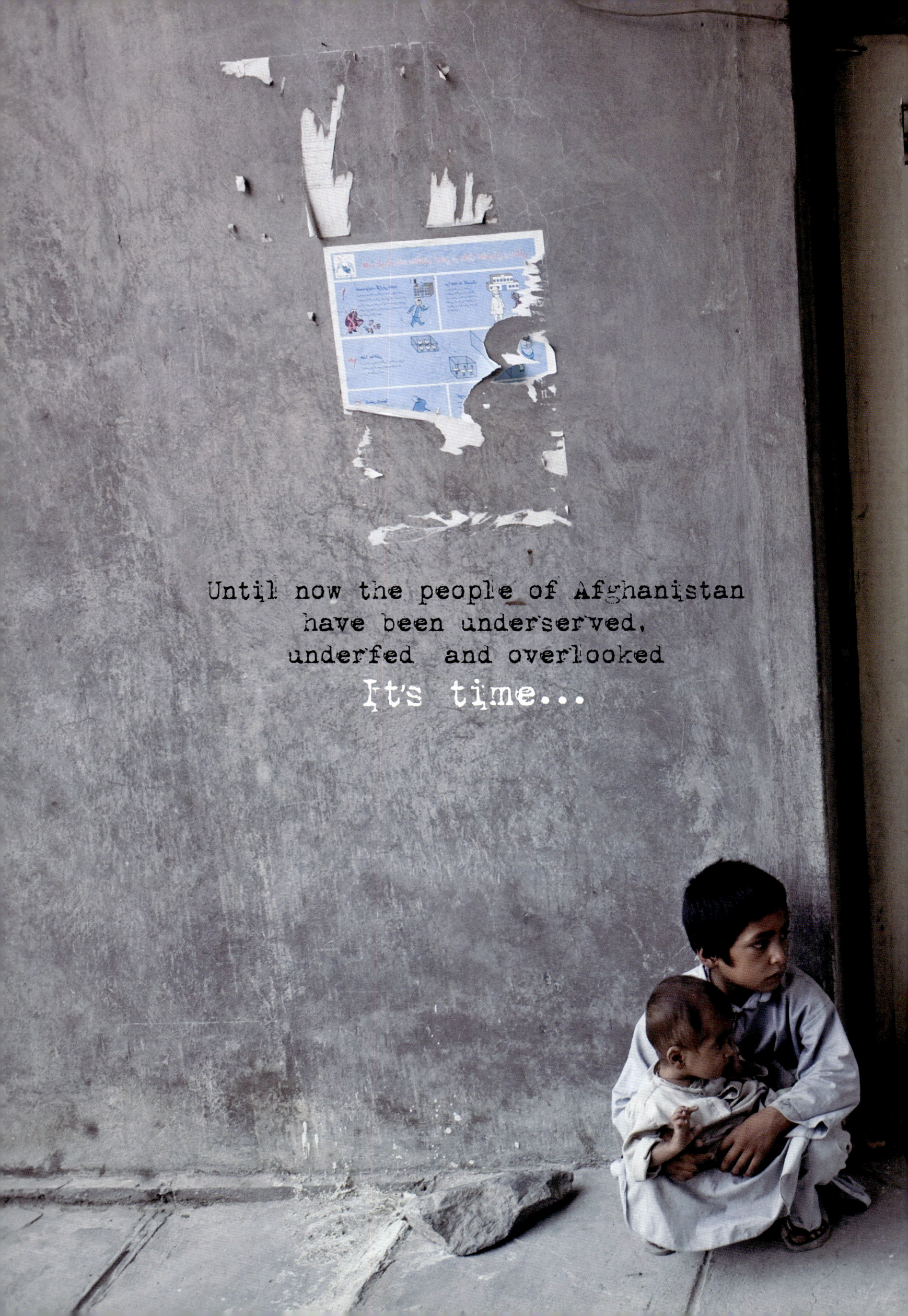

[Stop]

Tuberculosis in Afghanistan

by Anna Cataldi
Stop TB Ambassador and former UN Messenger of Peace

They come in their hundreds every morning (except Friday, which is the Holy day in Afghanistan), arriving in dribs and drabs to wait patiently for the Ali Abad orthopedic clinic, run by the International Red Cross in Kabul, to open. All suffering from some severe physical handicap, they are prepared to submit to any treatment that might restore the mobility they need to lead a more normal life. Injuries sustained in war, loss of limbs to landmines, accidents at work, the consequences of polio, scoliosis, arthritis, paralysis or simple malnutrition – these are the everyday problems in a country such as Afghanistan.

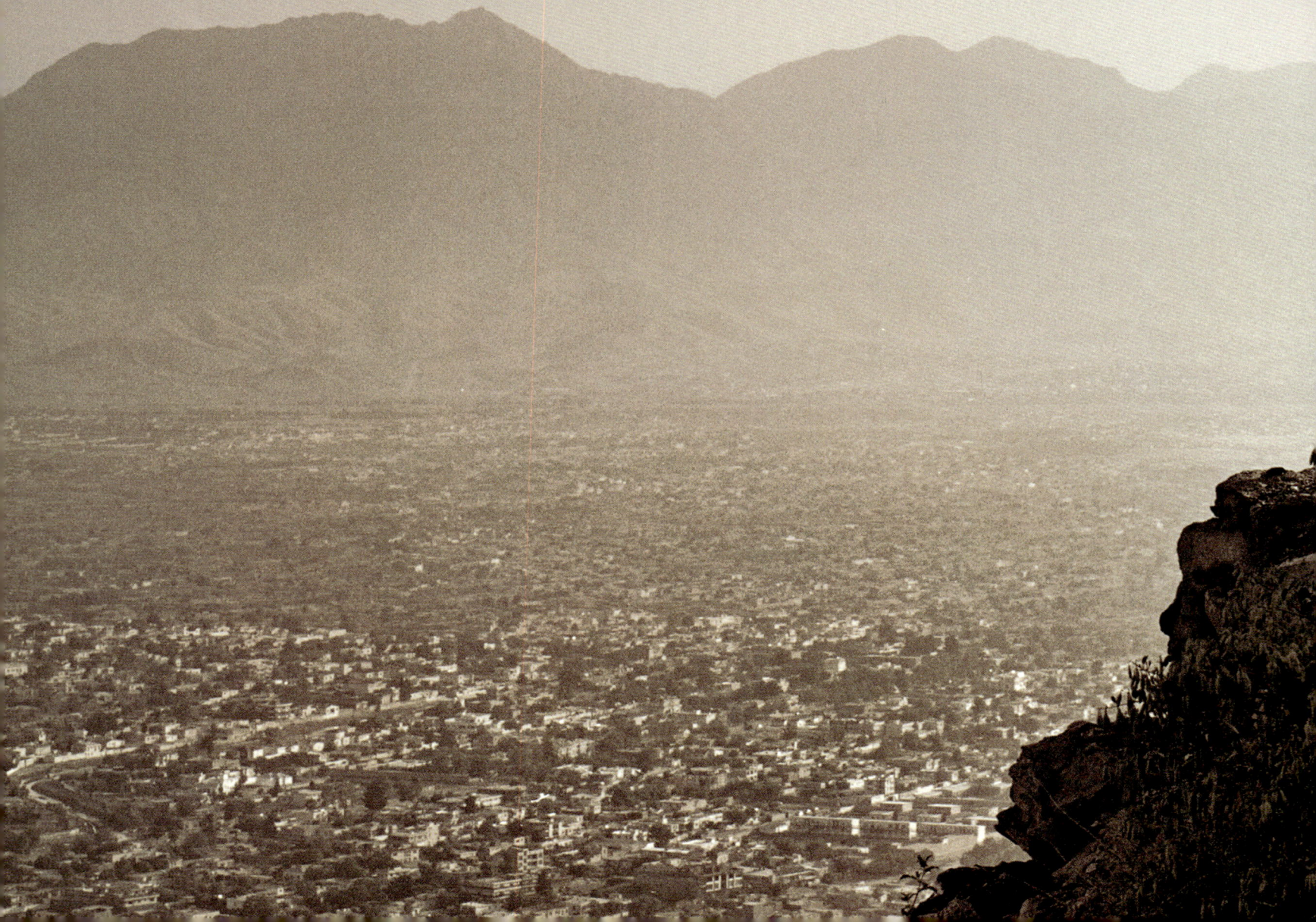

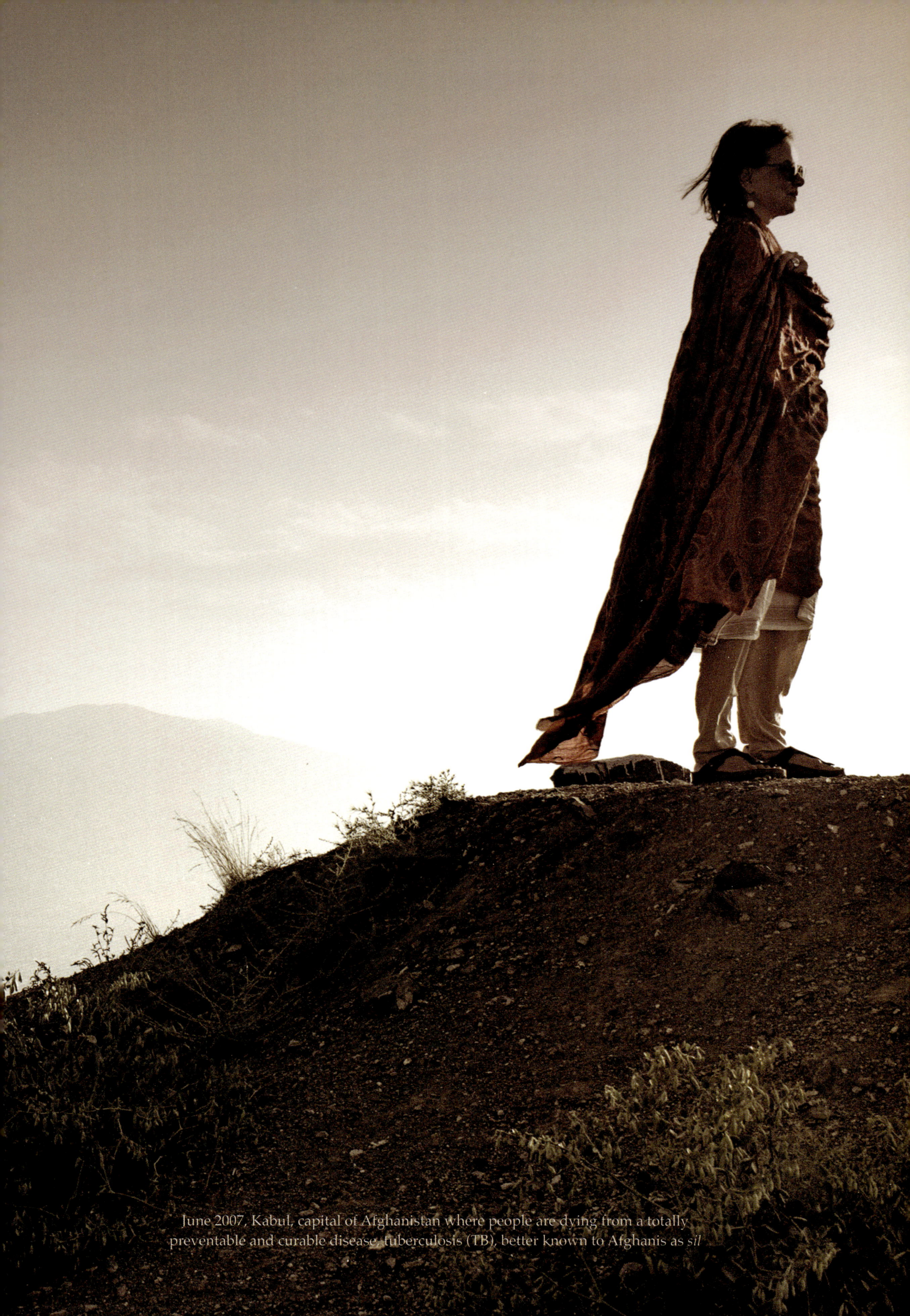

June 2007, Kabul, capital of Afghanistan where people are dying from a totally preventable and curable disease, tuberculosis (TB), better known to Afghanis as *sil*

Fazilla, a girl of 14, arrived on 19th May 2007. Her hospital number would be 33062. Her father, a tall, silent man, carried her in, cradling her gently in his arms. Her mother followed, shielding the wasted, pain-racked body of her child from accidental knocks. The pain came from sores caused by months spent practically immobile in bed, when every movement increased the suffering that was her only companion during the interminable hours, by day and night. No school, no sky, no sun, no clouds, nothing but the walls of the humble home in Yaka Tut, one of the poorest districts in Kabul. Until the age of ten, Fazilla had been a perfectly normal little girl, lively, active, a happy member of the numerous family comprising parents, grandparents, five brothers and a sister.

Then she began to complain of pain in her legs. Slowly, the pain, now excruciating, began creeping up to her back. Walking became more difficult every day. They took her to see the doctor. He diagnosed rheumatoid arthritis. This was in 2004. Despite the prescribed drugs, the painkillers and anti-inflammatories, the pain continued to intensify. Different prescriptions, more tests. X-rays revealed a serious scoliosis of the spine. In 2005, a team of foreign doctors, specialist pediatricians, carried out numerous tests at the Indira Gandhi hospital. They suspected a tumour, but this turned out not to be the case. Fazilla was sent home. She was now completely unable to walk. Her spine was so deformed that she was bent almost double. Even sitting was impossible.

In the summer of 2006 the condition was finally diagnosed: a very rare, insidious form of tuberculosis affecting the bones. Known to science as tubercular spondylitis, or Pott's Disease, it is notoriously difficult to diagnose.

It was at this point that she was put on the standard treatment already in use for a decade against all forms of TB. It consists of a cocktail of antibiotics effective against *Mycobacterium tuberculosis*, the micro-organism which was slowly sapping the child's life. The full course lasts for eight months, during which time the tablets have to be taken regularly every day, with no disruptions and extreme punctuality. Strict adherence to the prescribed schedule is the most important factor governing the efficacy of the cure.

In view of this, the World Health Organization (WHO) set up the Directly Observed Treatment Short-course (DOTS), providing for the strict monitoring of the therapy for optimum therapeutic benefit. Applied since 1995 to more than 26 million people in 187 different countries, DOTS has been responsible for the complete cure of the illness in 84% of cases. The total cost for 8 – 9 months of treatment? Twenty US dollars, less than 18 euros!!

When the course had been completed, Fazilla was tested again for TB. The result this time was negative. There was not a single trace of the dreaded *Mycobacterium tuberculosis* in her body.

Sadly, in spite of the cure there is no happy ending to report, because Fazilla's bones have been irreversibly damaged, especially during the very vulnerable growth stage of adolescence. The TB has been defeated, the degenerative process arrested, but the consequences remain. And the damage left behind in the wake of this unequal battle is devastating. Her spine, which will never be straight again, causes muscles to contract throughout the pathetically wasted body scarred as a result of the long time spent in bed.

At the Red Cross clinic they will do their best to help her, alleviating the pain with medicines and providing some rehabilitation therapy. Supported in a cradle of foam rubber cushions, Fazilla is very gently turned almost every hour. Little by little the lesions will heal. Fed on a very high-calorie diet – five meals a day – she will eventually regain that modicum of energy necessary for attempting the first gentle physiotherapy exercises. Perhaps, if things go well, she will be able to sit with the help of a brace and walk a few steps supported by a Zimmer frame. But the future for this girl with her sensitive face and dark, deep-set eyes bright with intelligence is already marked out. No man, in a country as poor as Afghanistan, would dream of marrying a woman this badly handicapped who could be of no help in the home.

A smile lights up Fazilla's face when they talk to her about resuming her studies. As a bedridden invalid, she lost three years of schooling. She dreams about learning English. Here at the centre there are teachers ready to help her, but at home, how can she possibly attend school? Sad enough already, Fazilla's case is even sadder when one considers that had her TB been diagnosed from the start she could have been completely cured in a matter of months with very little expense and no need for hospitalization. The fact is that it is now possible not only to control TB but to cure it. Unlike AIDS, for example, which can be controlled by the new drugs but never cured.

As old as the history of man himself (the genome of TB has been found in Egyptian mummies) but easily recognizable despite its various names and the diverse cultures in which appeared throughout the centuries TB was an almost inevitable sentence of death for whoever contracted the disease. Then one day in March 1882 an obscure German doctor's report that in the course of his experiments he had succeeded in discovering the hitherto unknown cause of the disease, immediately revolutionized the history of TB.

By producing proof that the cause of Tuberculosis was a specific microscopic bacillus (*Mycobacterium tuberculosis*) this doctor, Robert Koch, made diagnosis possible and laid the foundations of a therapeutic approach that only a few decades later would enable the medical profession to treat a disease against which mankind had been powerless for thousands of years.

In spite of this, nearly two million people still die from TB every year. The figure quoted by the WHO is one million eight hundred thousand or five thousand a day. Imagine reading in the paper day after day that 15 planes each carrying 300 people had crashed with no survivors. More devastating than malaria, which affects only countries plagued by mosquitoes, TB – spread not through direct contact but by airborne droplets – can infect anyone anywhere.

Data provided by the WHO also show that two billion people – one third of the world's population – have been infected by the TB bacillus. Not all of them become ill, however. In nine cases out of ten the bacillus remains latent and causes no problems. But in the case of a weakened immune system – the populations of Third-World countries are the most vulnerable because TB, AIDS and poverty go hand in hand – then the bacillus becomes active, attacks the host body and causes the disease. The most common form is TB of the lungs, or pulmonary TB. In Afghanistan they call it «sill». The immediately recognizable symptoms are a cough accompanied by the spitting of blood.

Ten years ago Zakayeva, a Hazara woman of 25 pregnant with her fifth child while still breast-feeding the fourth, watched her mother die of TB. Even before the cough started to rack her own chest she was in no doubt whatsoever about the disease that was making her feel so tired she could not stand, that was drenching her body with sweat and inducing icy shivers.

Zakayeva's family lives in extreme poverty even by the standards of Afghanistan, a country that is one of the poorest of the poor. The irregular earnings of her husband, a builder dependent on piece-work, are frequently insufficient to feed the four children, his wife and himself and an old, sick grandfather who all live crowded into a single room almost always in deep darkness. Even on sunny days no light manages to penetrate the gloom from the single north-facing window. In spite of all this, Zakayeva's smile was sweetness itself as, cradling her latest-born in her arms, she said that from the day she began her TB treatment things had – thanks be to God – improved, she no longer suffered from headaches and felt less tired. She receives her tablets free from the WHO and her treatment card entitles her to receive a sack of rice and a can of oil every month. These supplementary rations are provided by the World Food Programme (WFP) which, because malnutrition is so often the root cause of the disease, collaborates with the WHO in the fight against TB.

One has to wonder how much of this food will benefit Zakayeva herself. Afghan women, like those in other Asian countries, having cooked the food will eat only the remains of the meal when all the others, primarily the men, have finished.

One of the statistical records held by Afghanistan is that here, as opposed to most of the rest of the world, women can expect to die earlier than men. Besides which, the percentage of women who succumb to TB is far higher than that of men. According to Dr Kakar, the Afghan Deputy Minister of Public Health, the two facts are related. Sexual discrimination forces women to live practically as recluses in homes that nearly always lack adequate ventilation, are overcrowded and walls often unhealthy. If you add the irritating effect on the lungs of smoke from the coal used for cooking, it is only too easy to understand why a person already weakened by malnutrition becomes a victim of diseases, among which TB predominates.

Fortunately the situation in Afghanistan has improved over the last three or four years. According to information released by the Ministry of Health, out of the 44% of TB patients monitored by the DOTS system, 89% have been completely cured.

Zakayeva will be cured and will give birth to a healthy child. The other members of her family stand a good chance of escaping infection, too, because even after the first month of treatment, TB ceases to be contagious. Not everyone, however, will be so lucky, especially in the years to come. This is what worries Dr Karam Shah, who, having organized the TB programme in Pakistan has been sent by the WHO to do to a similar job in Afghanistan. «At the moment,» he says, «the fight against TB, as is the case with other diseases, is producing a good rate of success. In Kabul the situation in the hospitals, doctors' surgeries and clinics has improved enormously in comparison with past years. The problem is that all this improvement is due solely to the humanitarian organizations and the funding Afghanistan receives from abroad. This makes for a situation that is fragile and unsustainable in the long term. Like a patient kept alive by oxygen who, as soon as the supply is switched off, will inevitably die.»

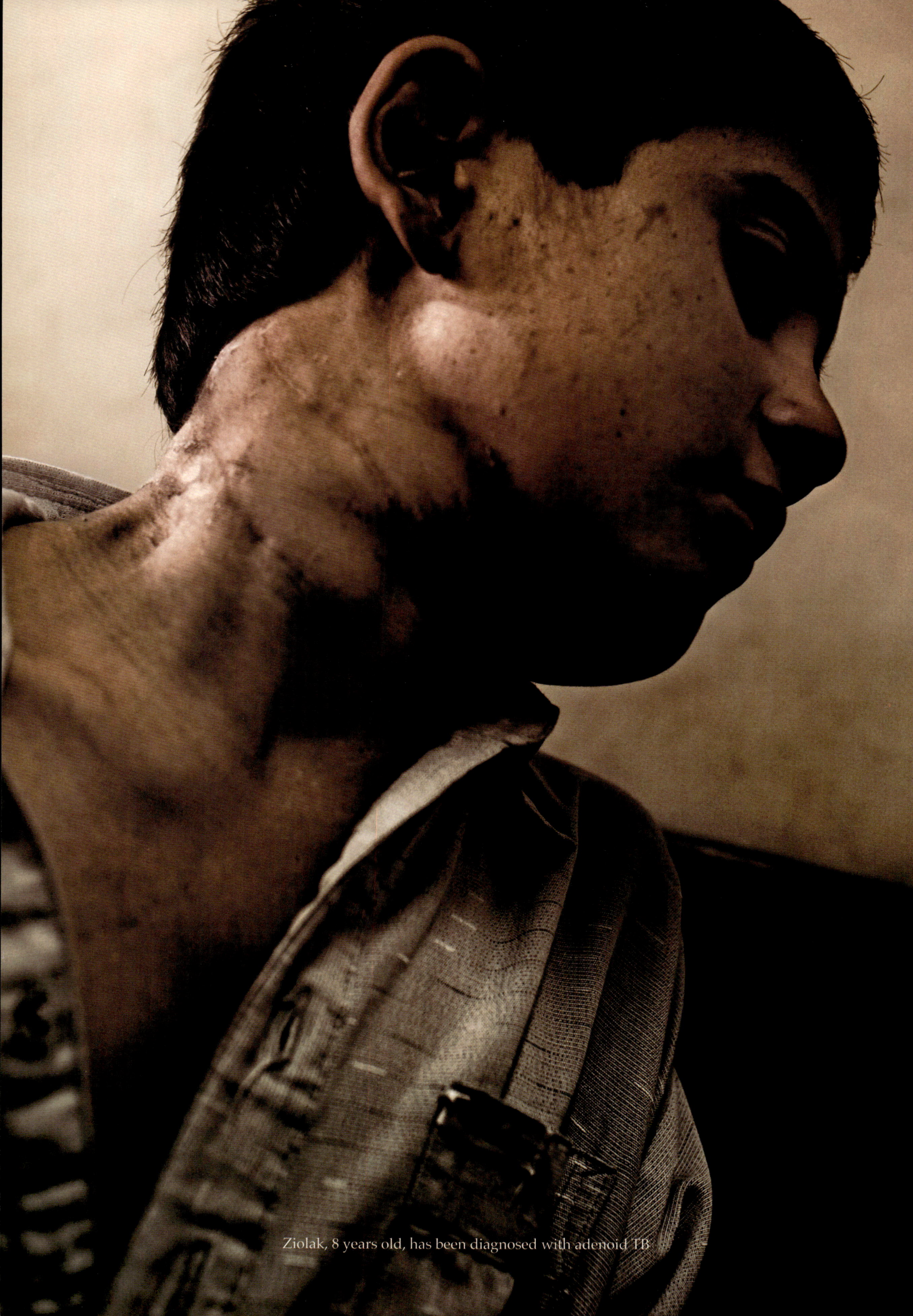
Ziolak, 8 years old, has been diagnosed with adenoid TB

All that is required to cure this deadly disease is
a simple treatment

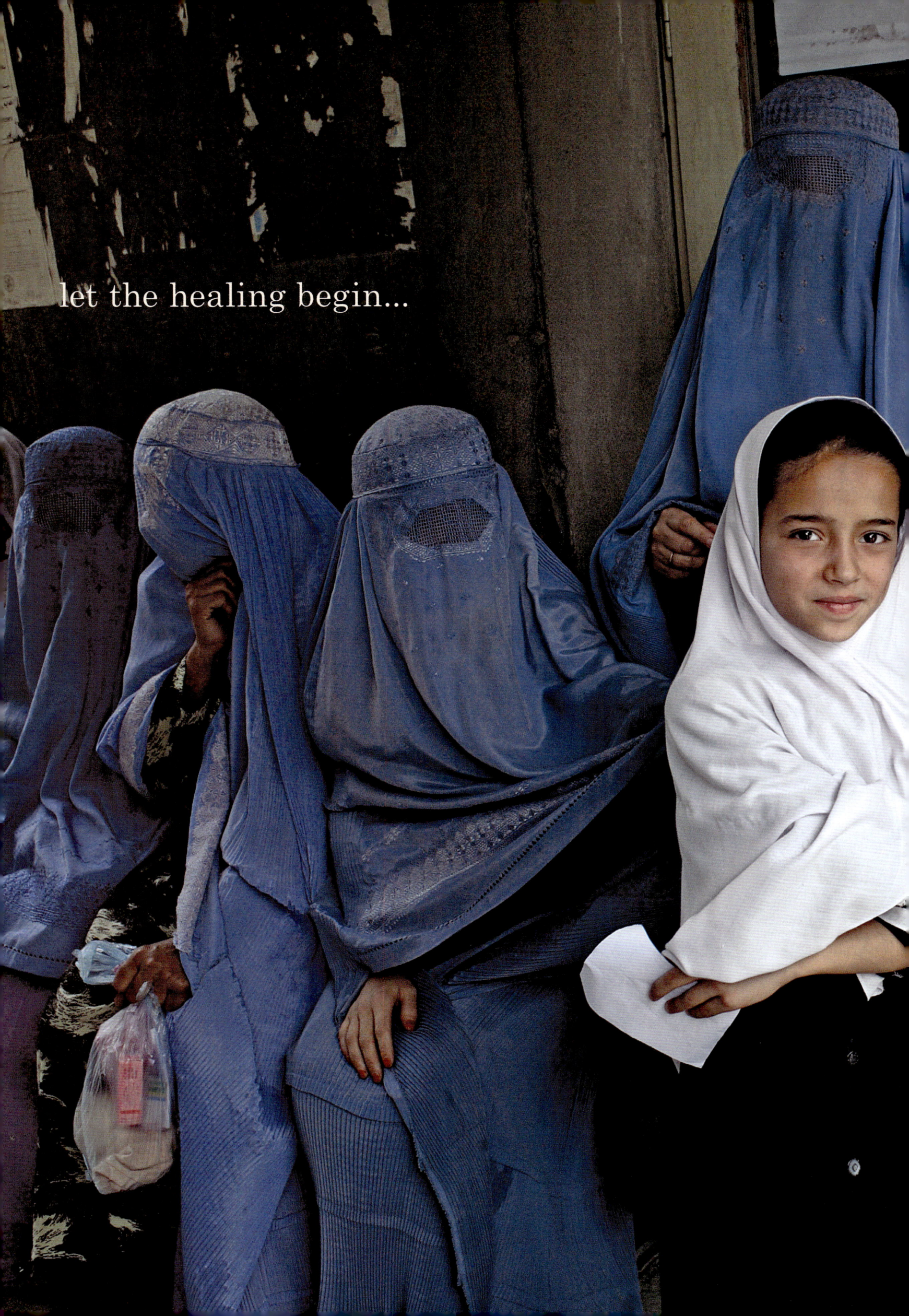

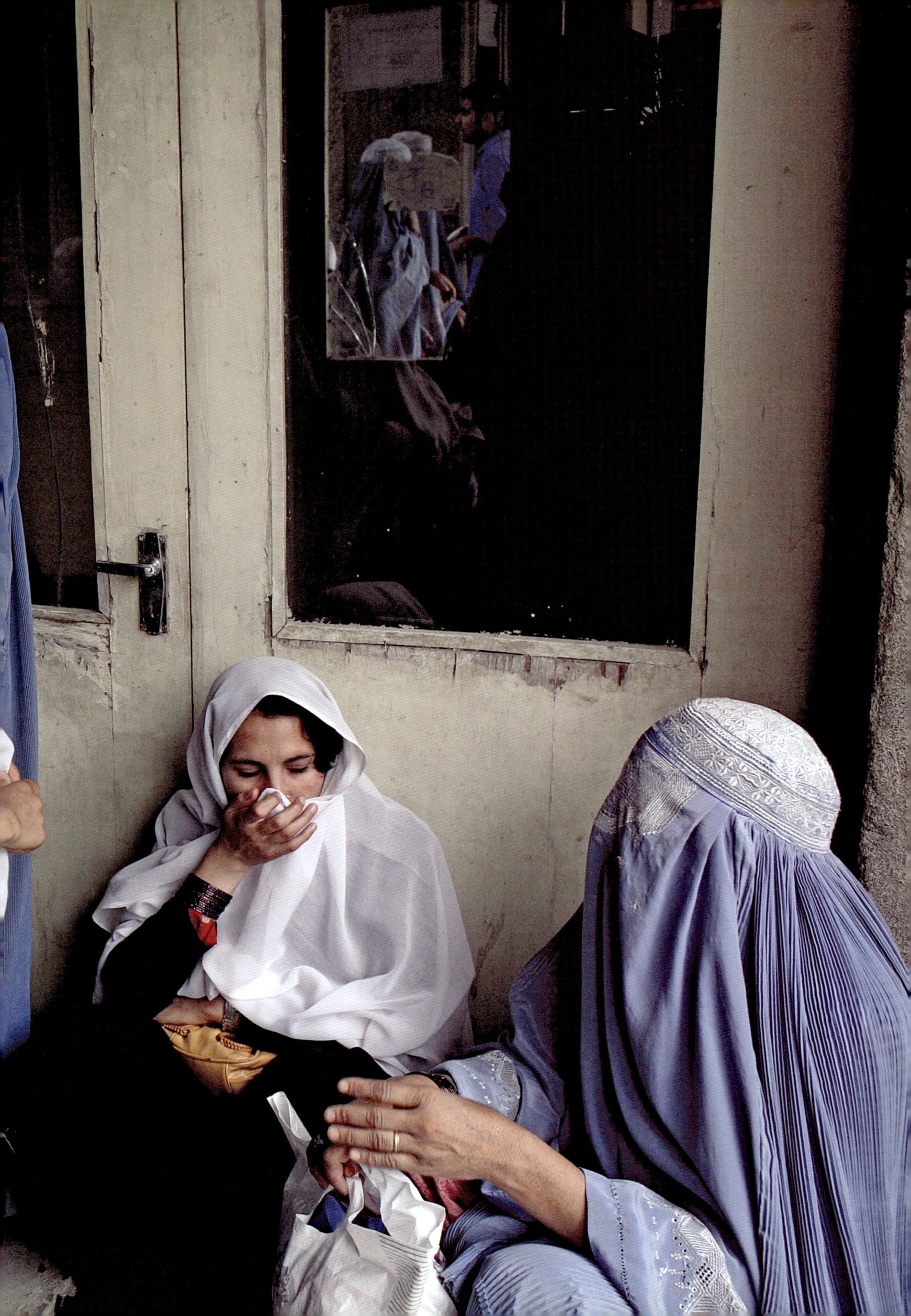

The first step towards
finding a solution is

acknowledging the existence of a problem

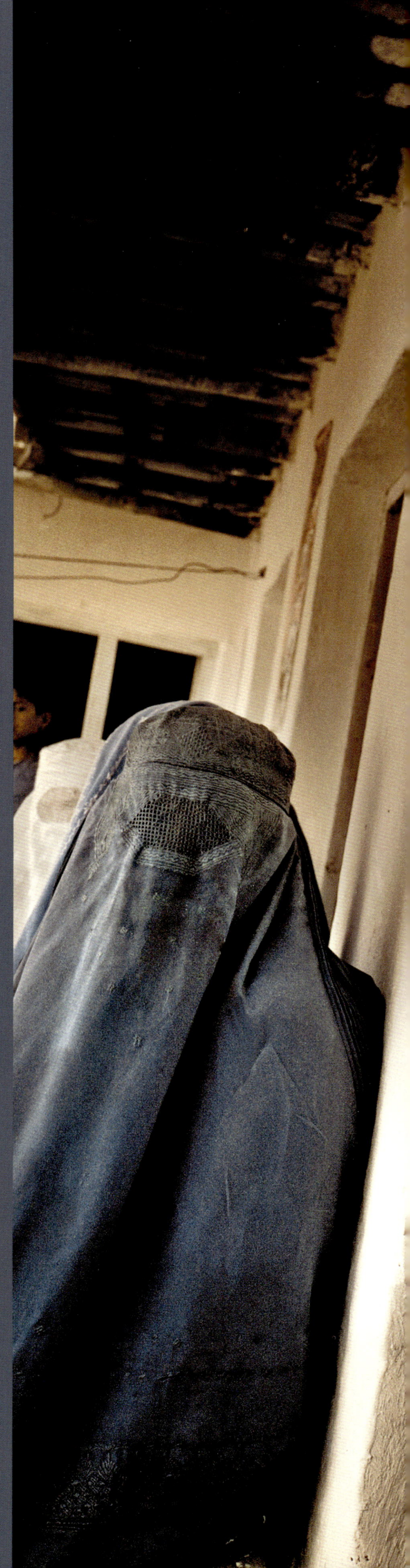

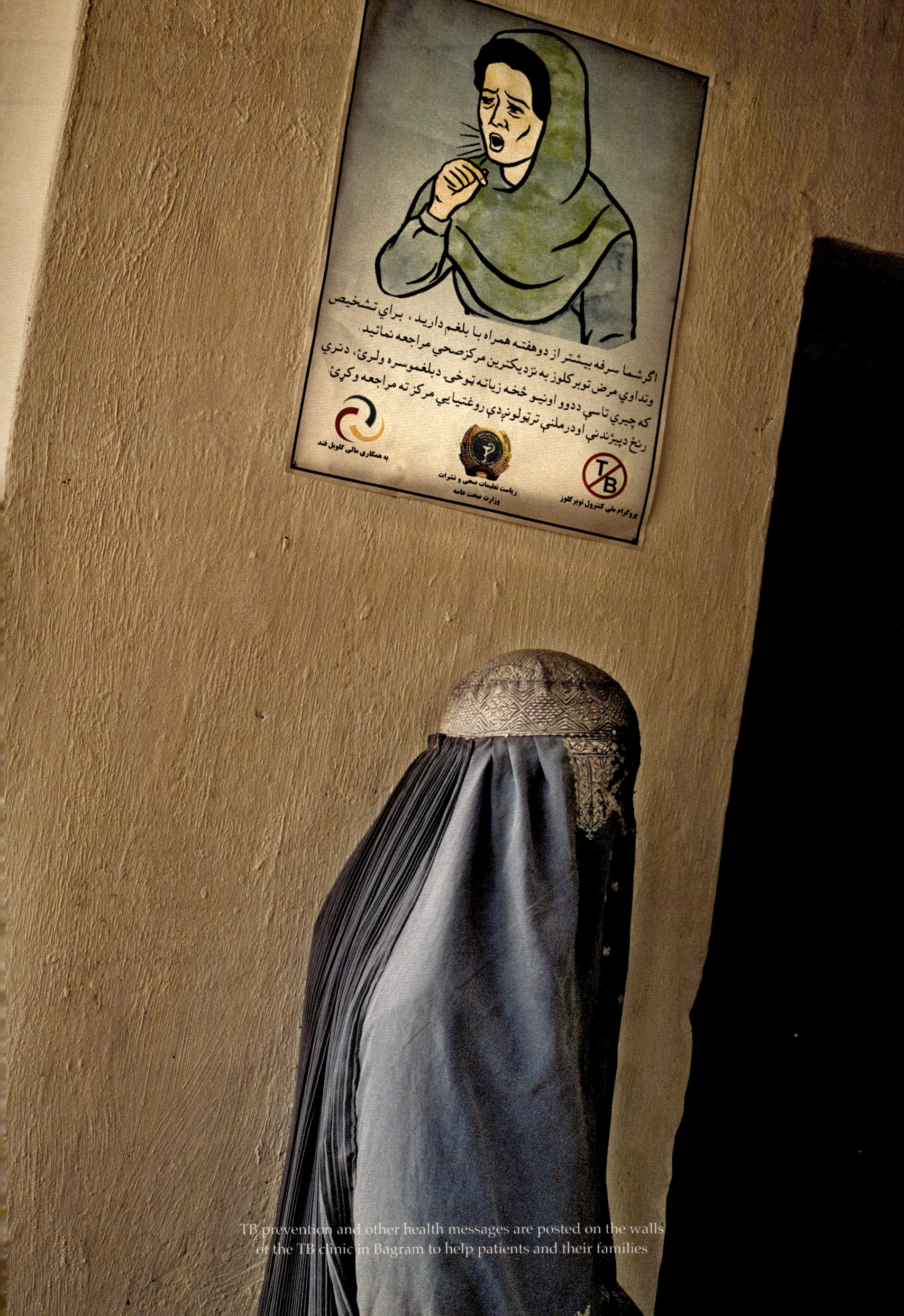

TB prevention and other health messages are posted on the walls of the TB clinic in Bagram to help patients and their families

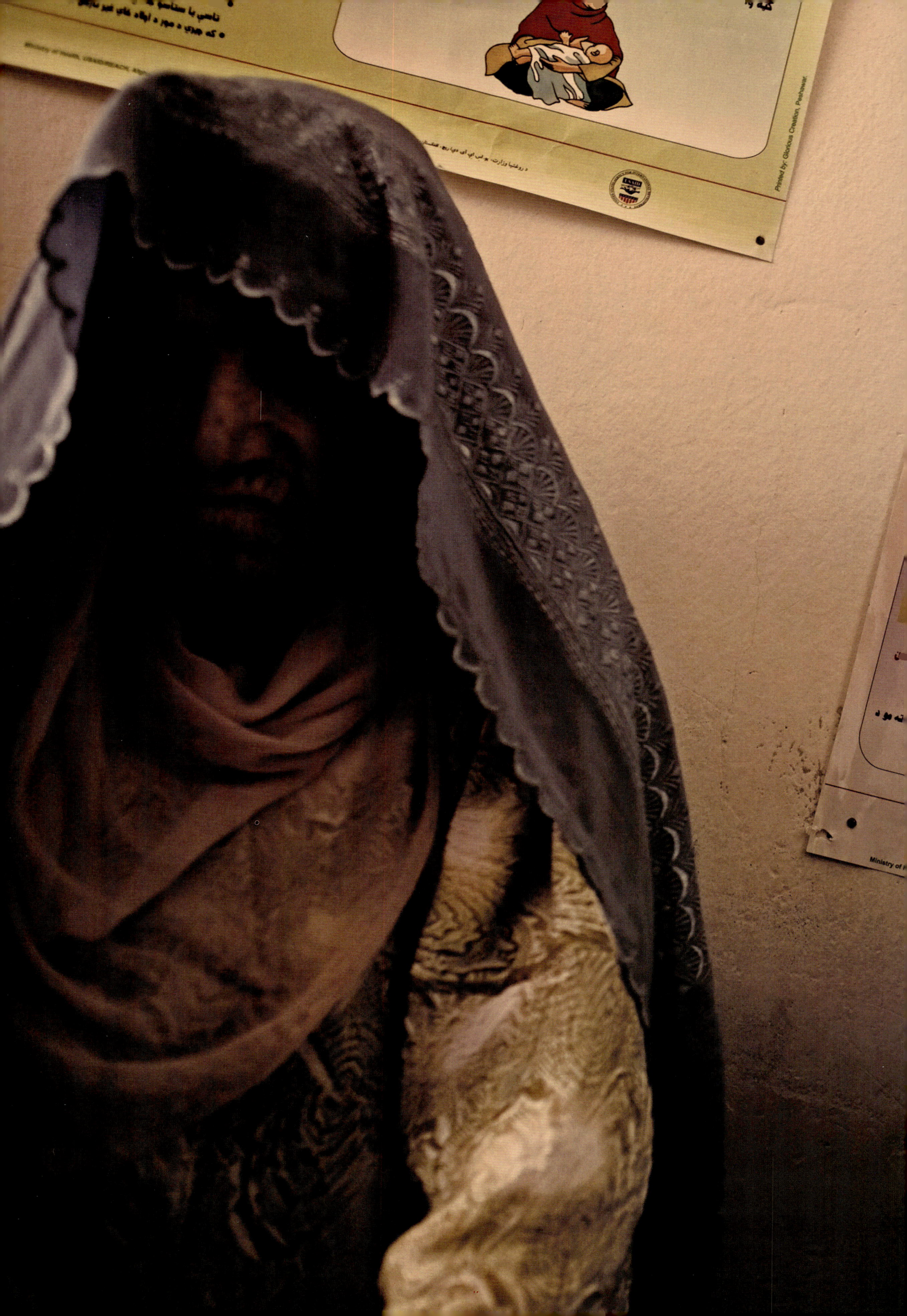

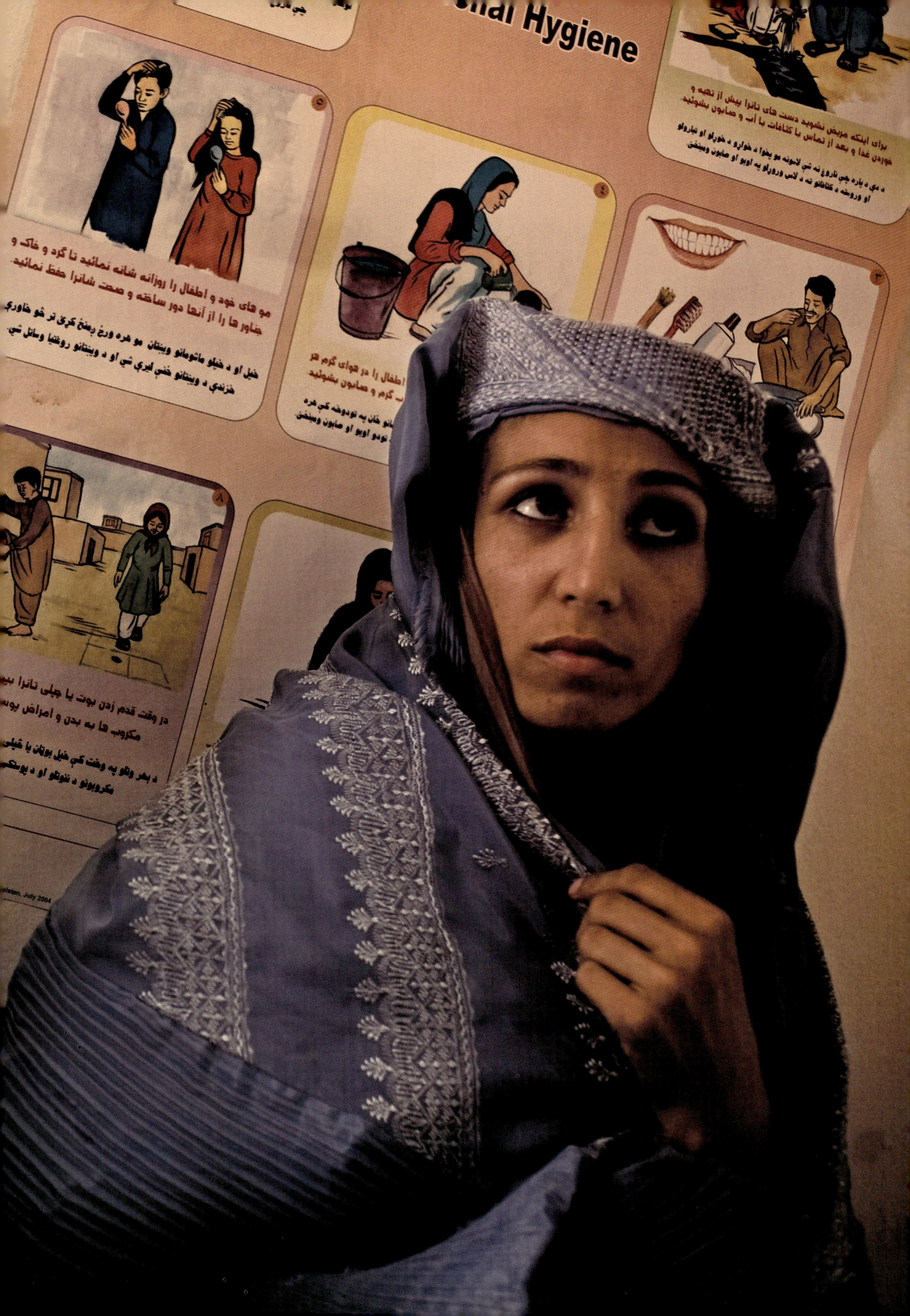

Proper investigation relies on
patience, expertise and understanding

National Tuberc...

Type of TB	Sex	DOTs	
Pulmonary Smear Positive	Male	7	
	Female	10	
	Children	1	1
Pulmonary Smear Negative	Male	2	4
	Femal	2	10
	children	4	3
Extra Pulmonary	Male	3	6
	Female	7	7
	Children	2	3
Total	Male	12	17
	Female	19	25
	Children	7	7
Total Grant		38	

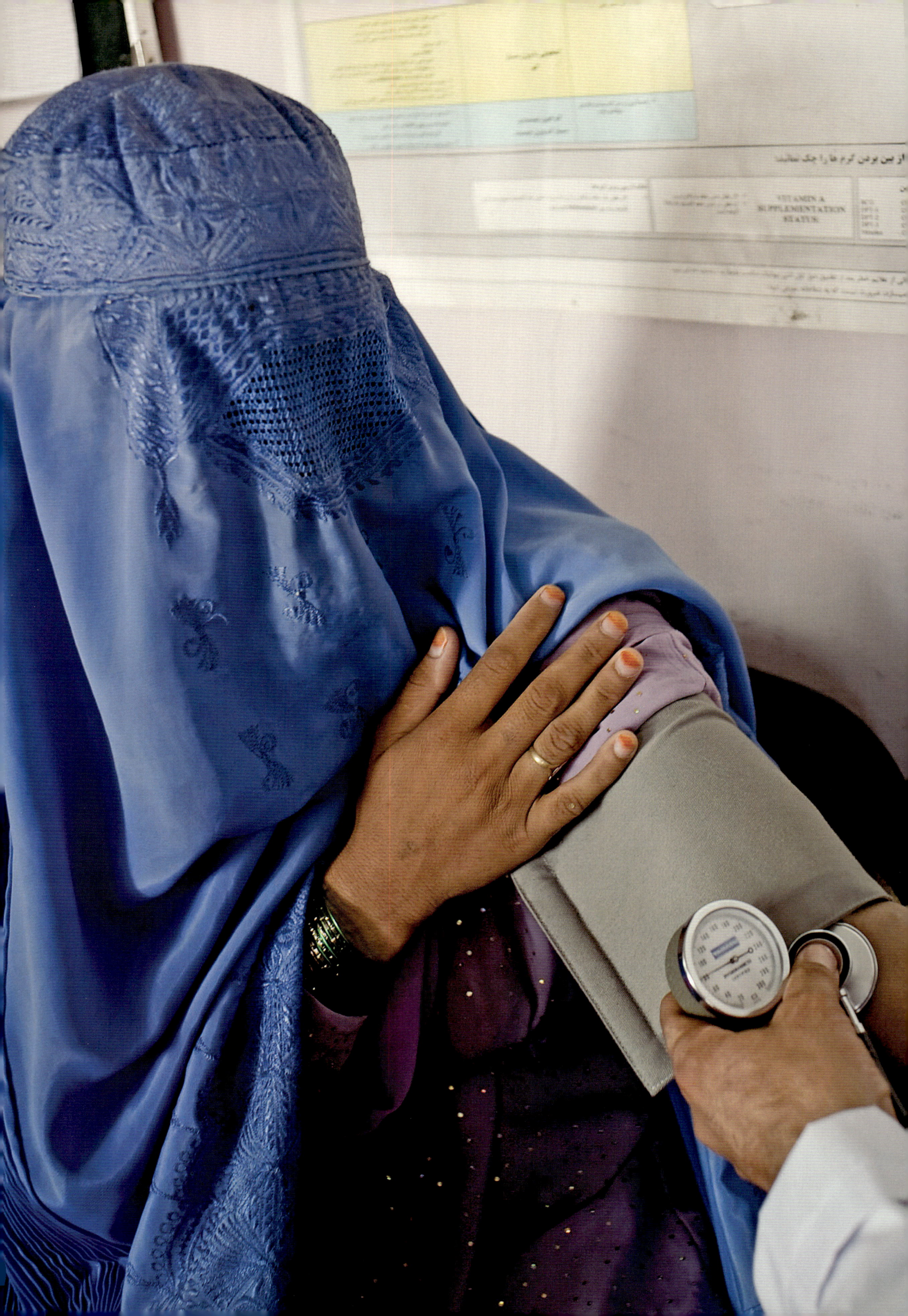

This woman is suspected to have TB and has come to the health post for examination

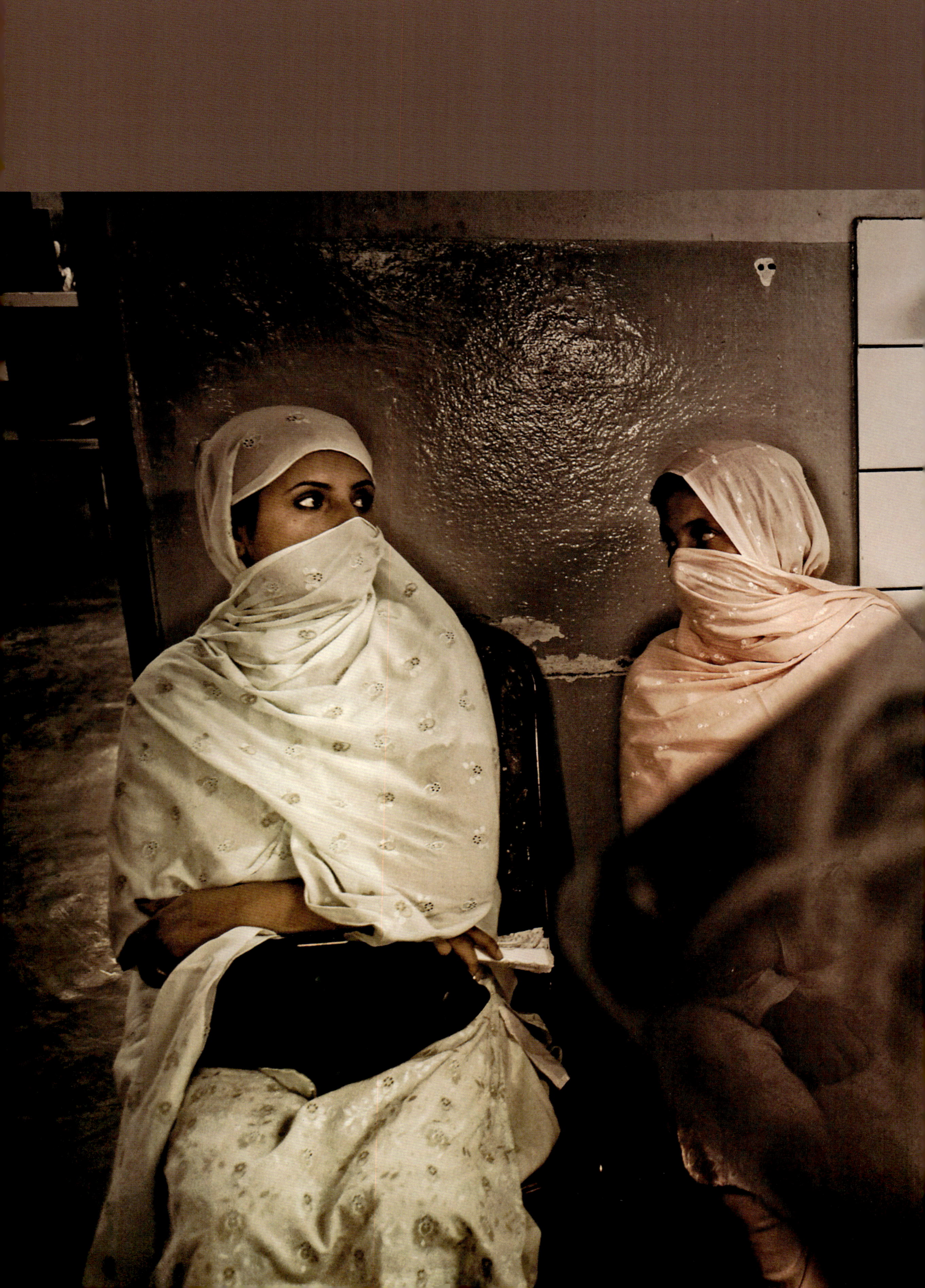

Proper attentiveness, proper analysis, proper identification and finally

proper conclusion

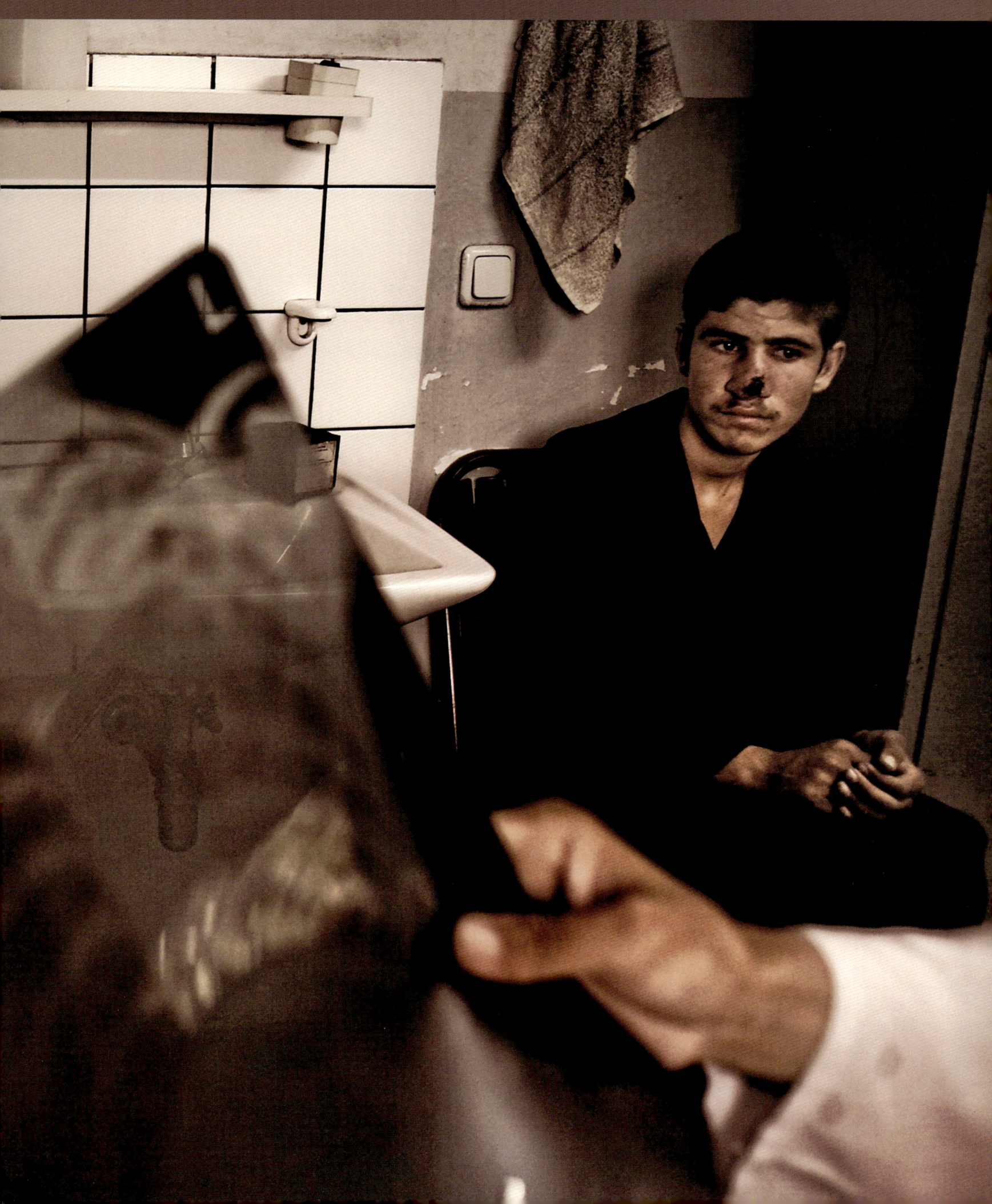

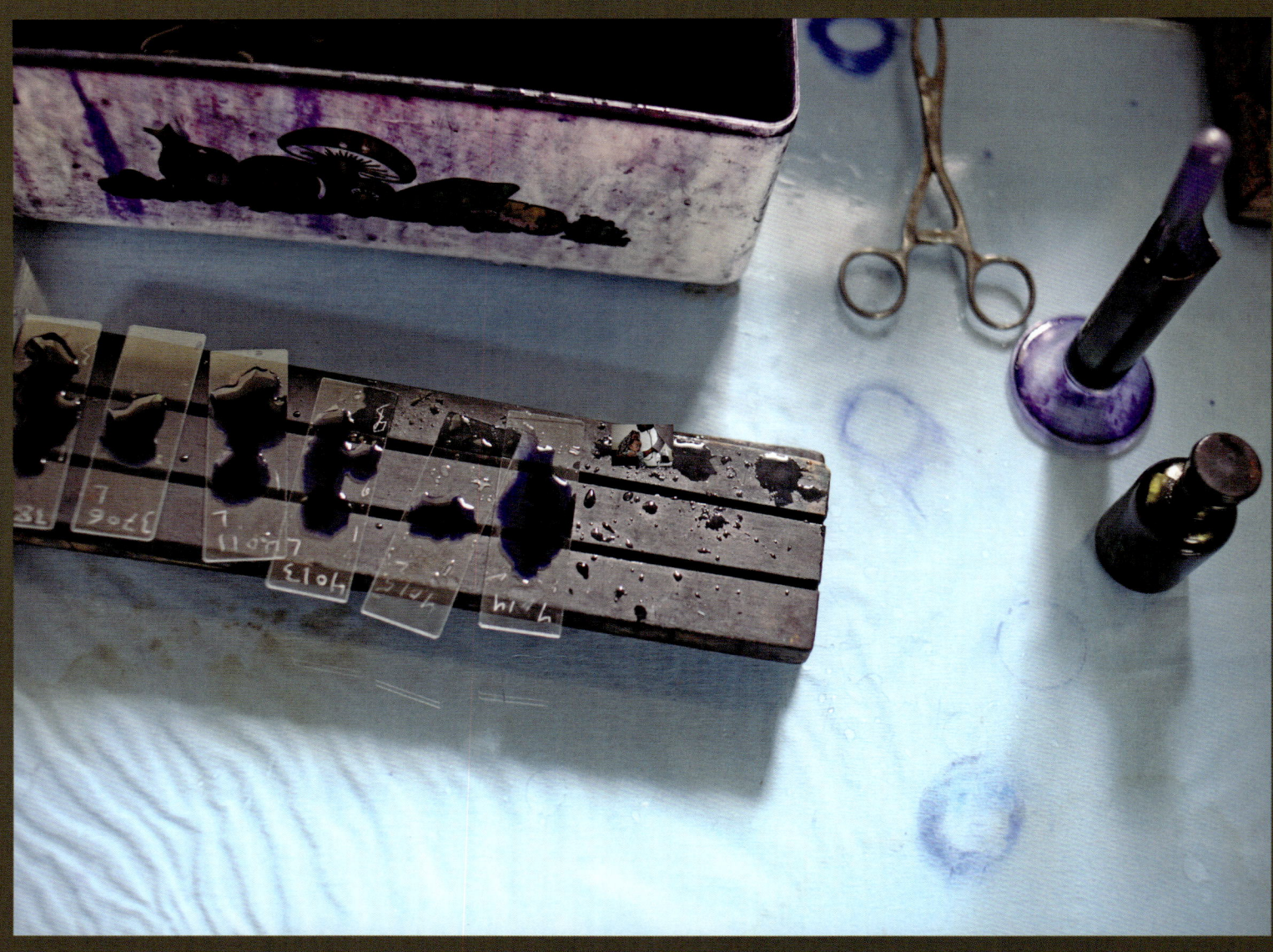

If laboratory results are positive for TB, the patient is immediately put on DOTS therapy

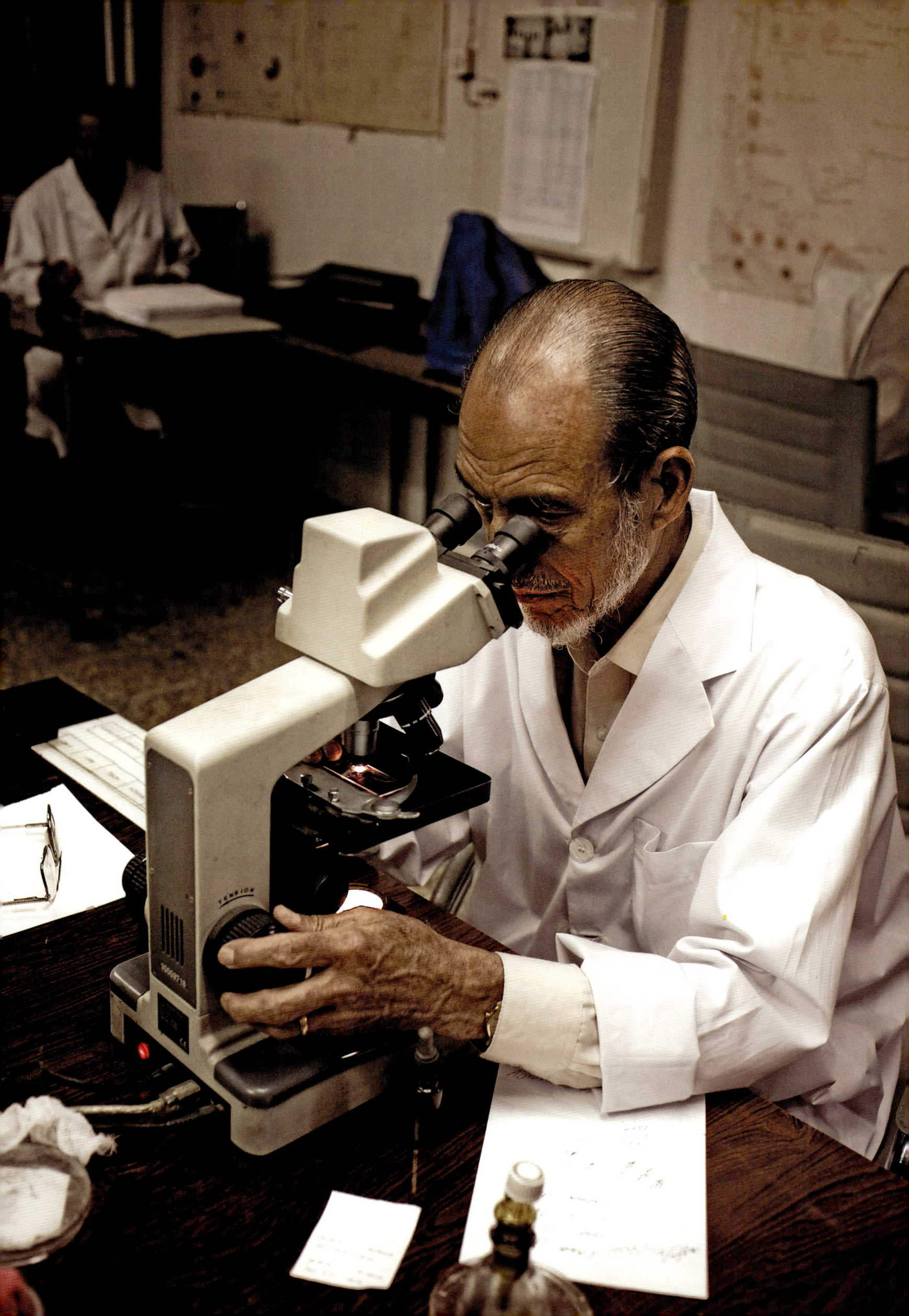

What is often seen as torment,
in this case is seen as hope

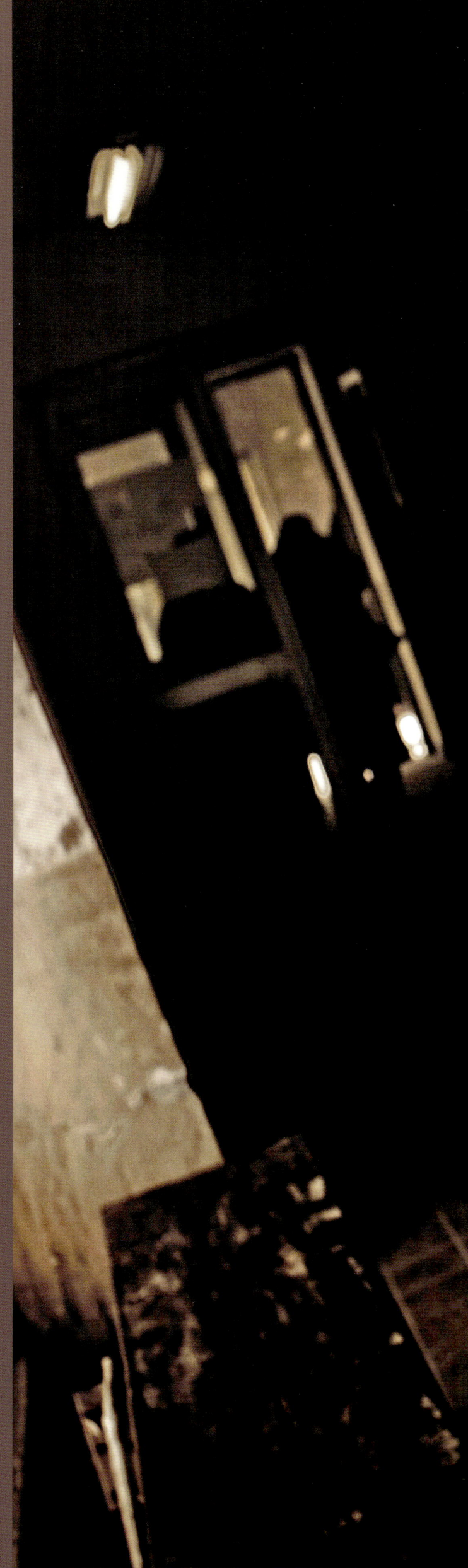

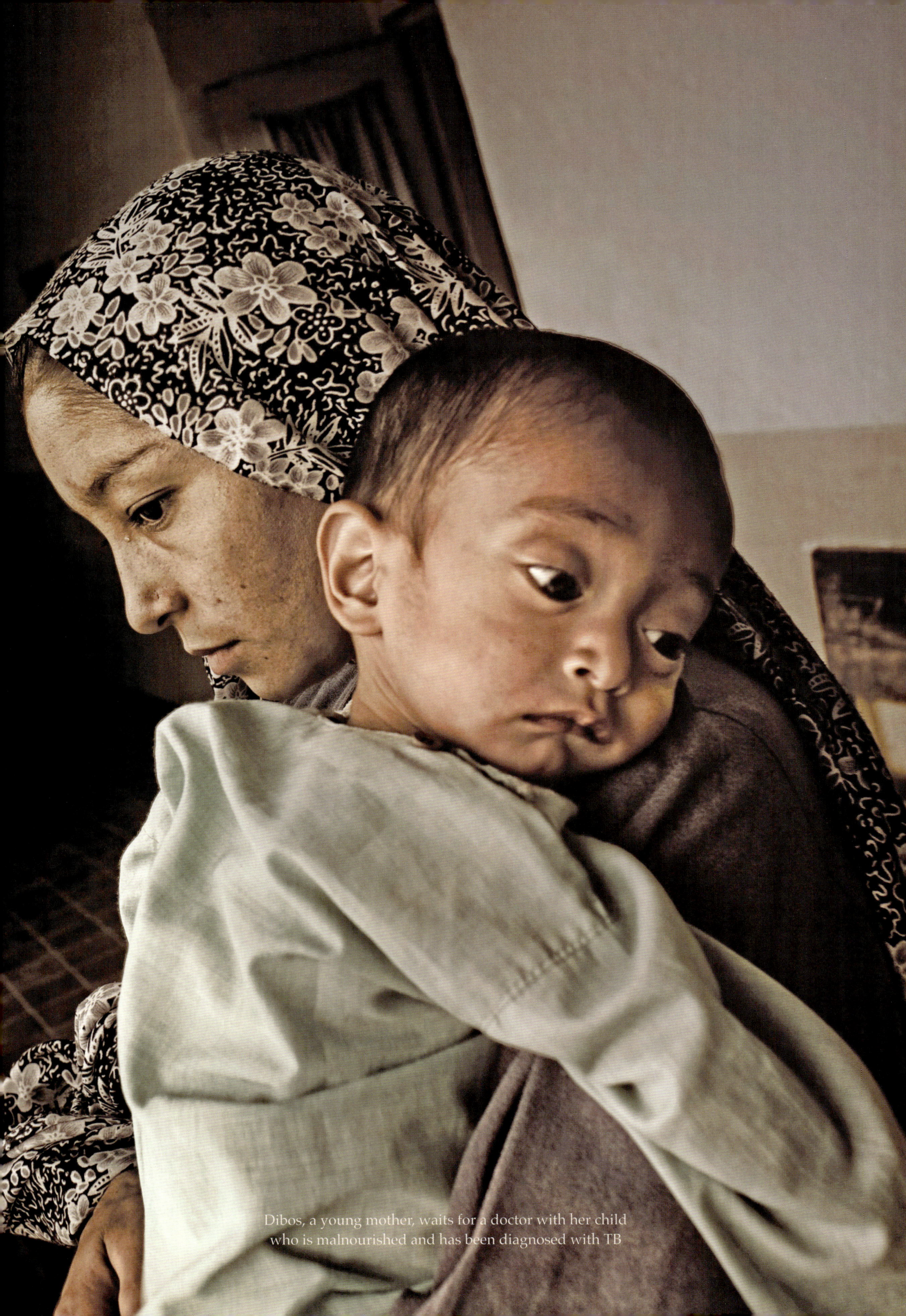

Dibos, a young mother, waits for a doctor with her child who is malnourished and has been diagnosed with TB

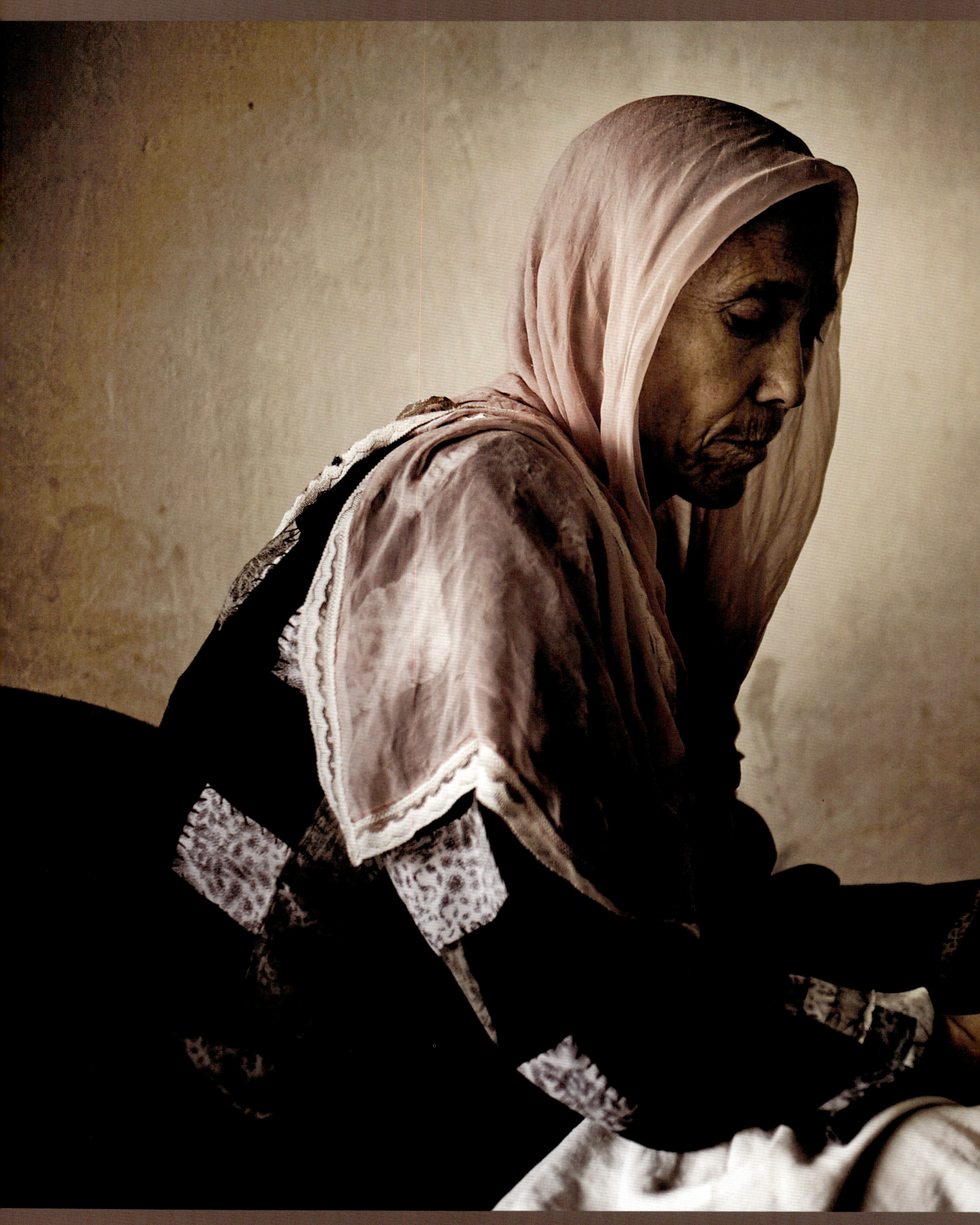
Vidorga, 33 years old, has been suffering from TB for the past 3 years but recently started receiving tuberculosis treatment

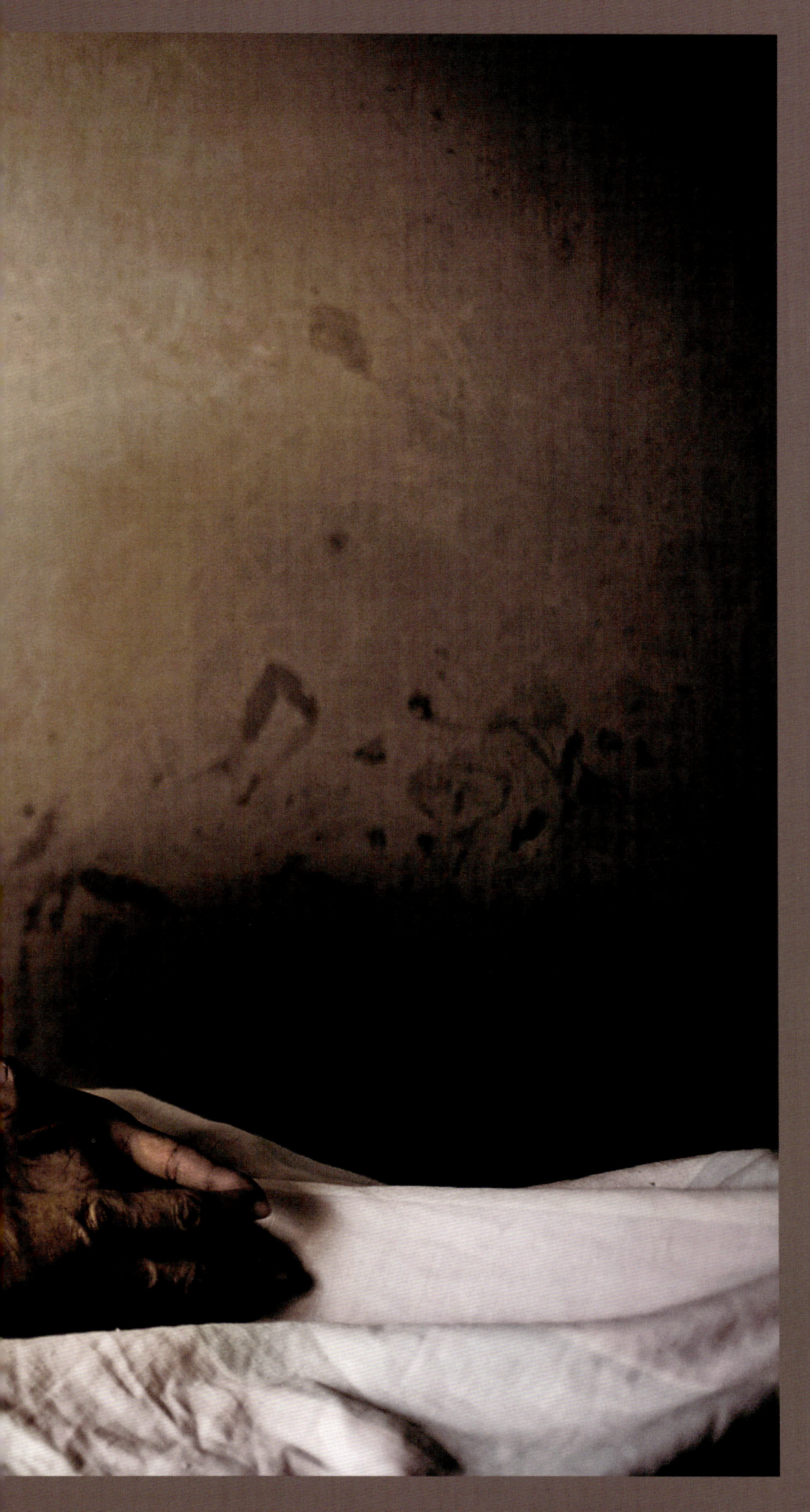

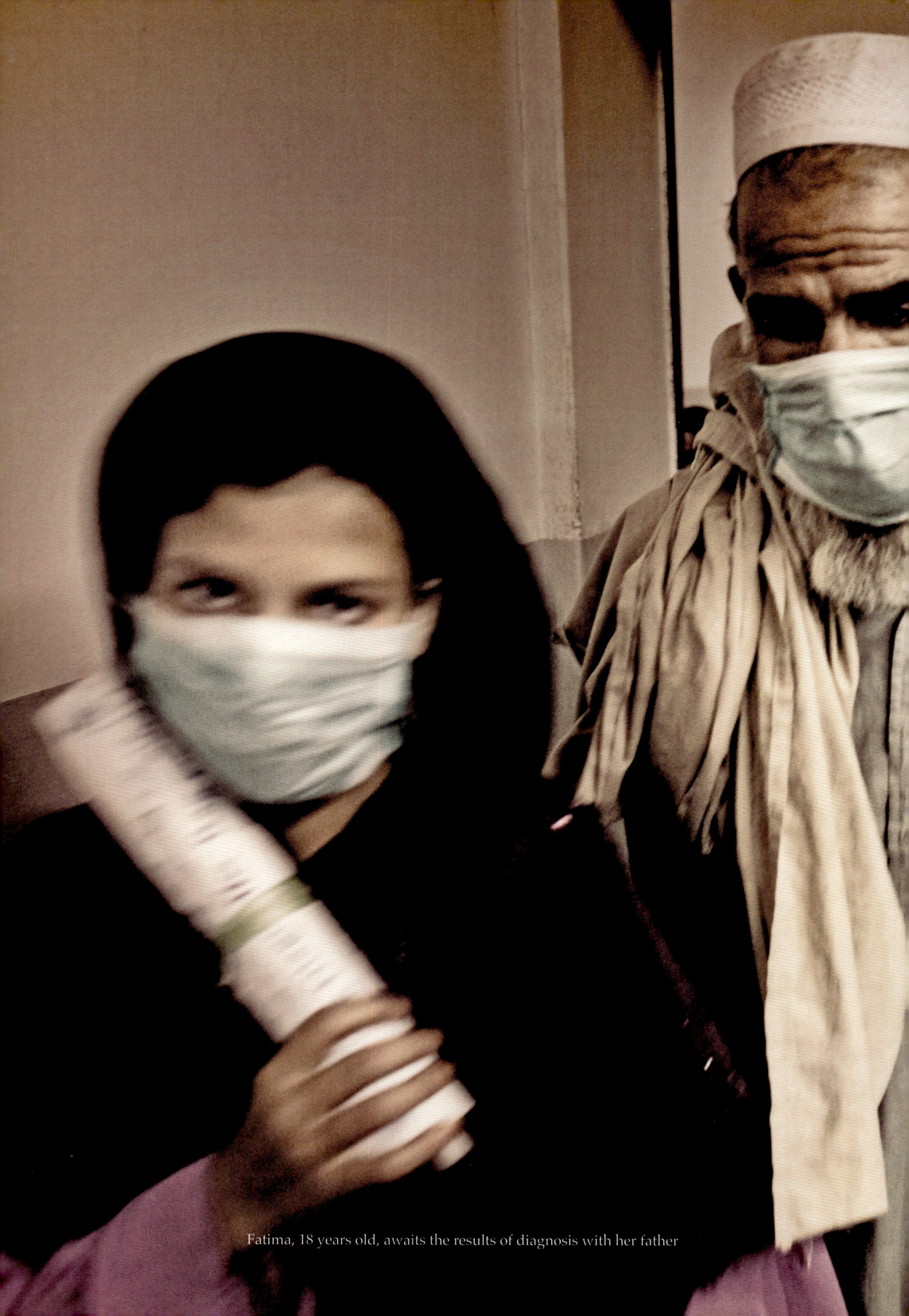

Fatima, 18 years old, awaits the results of diagnosis with her father

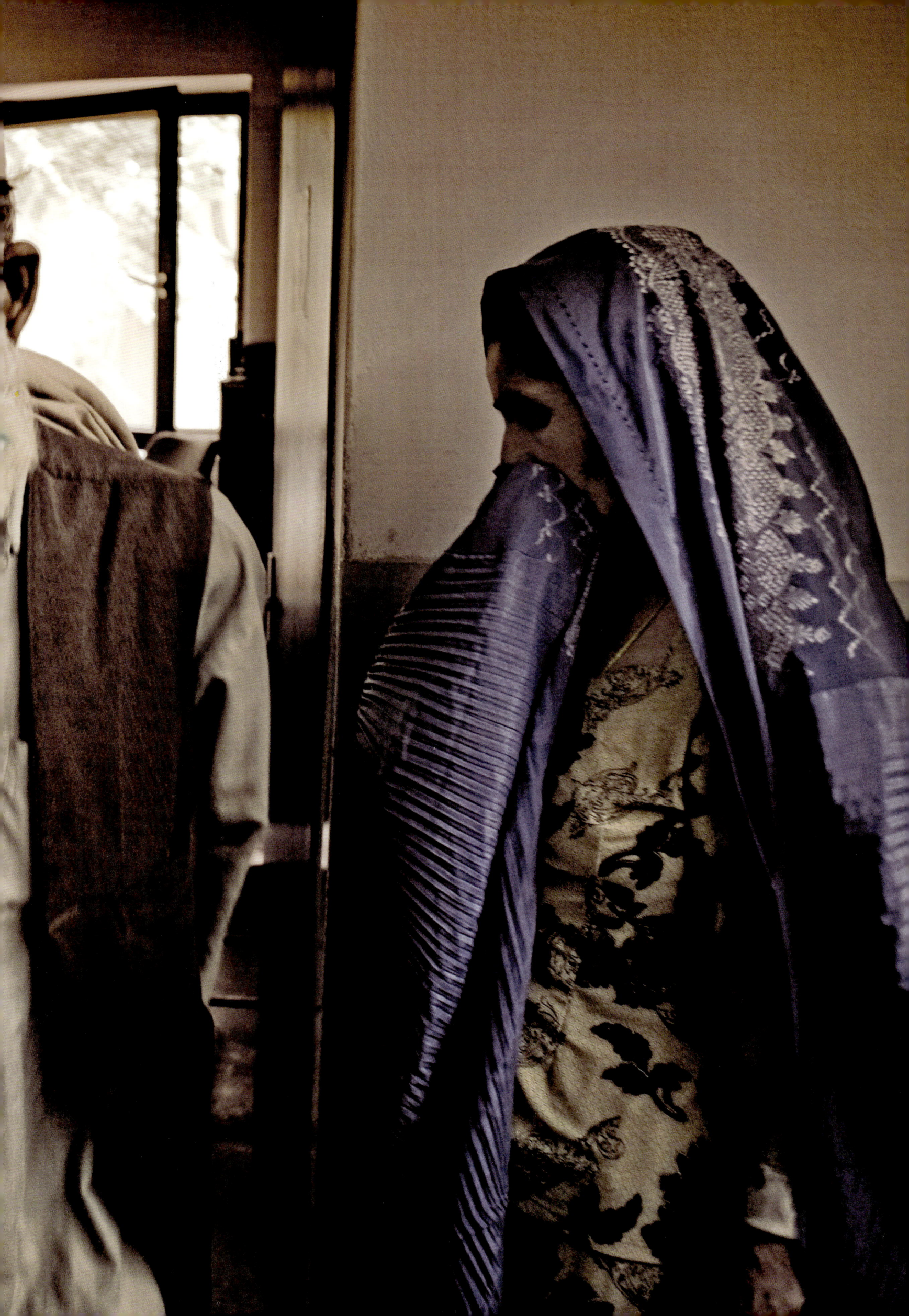

Sultan, 62 years old, is under treatment for drug-resistant TB

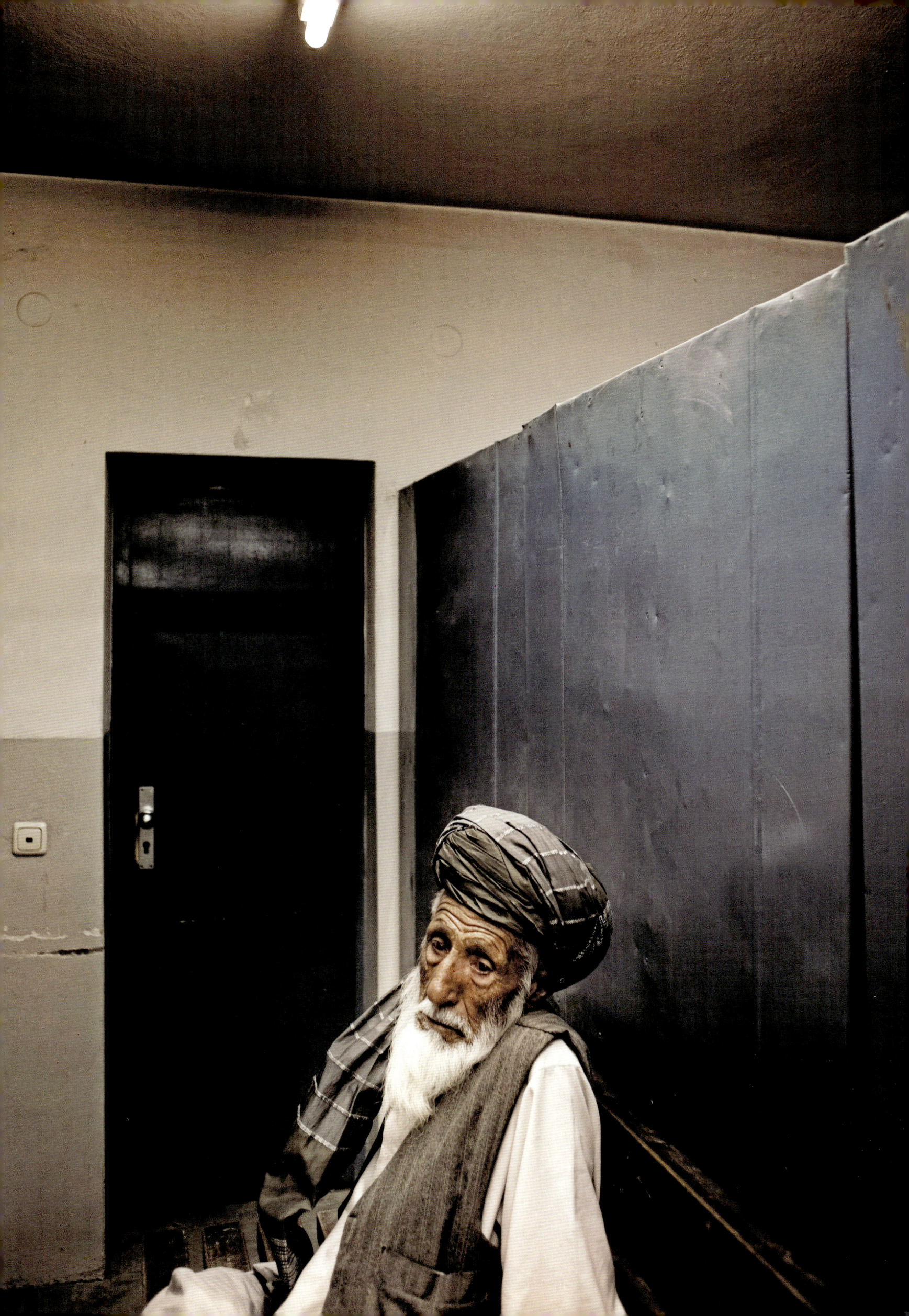

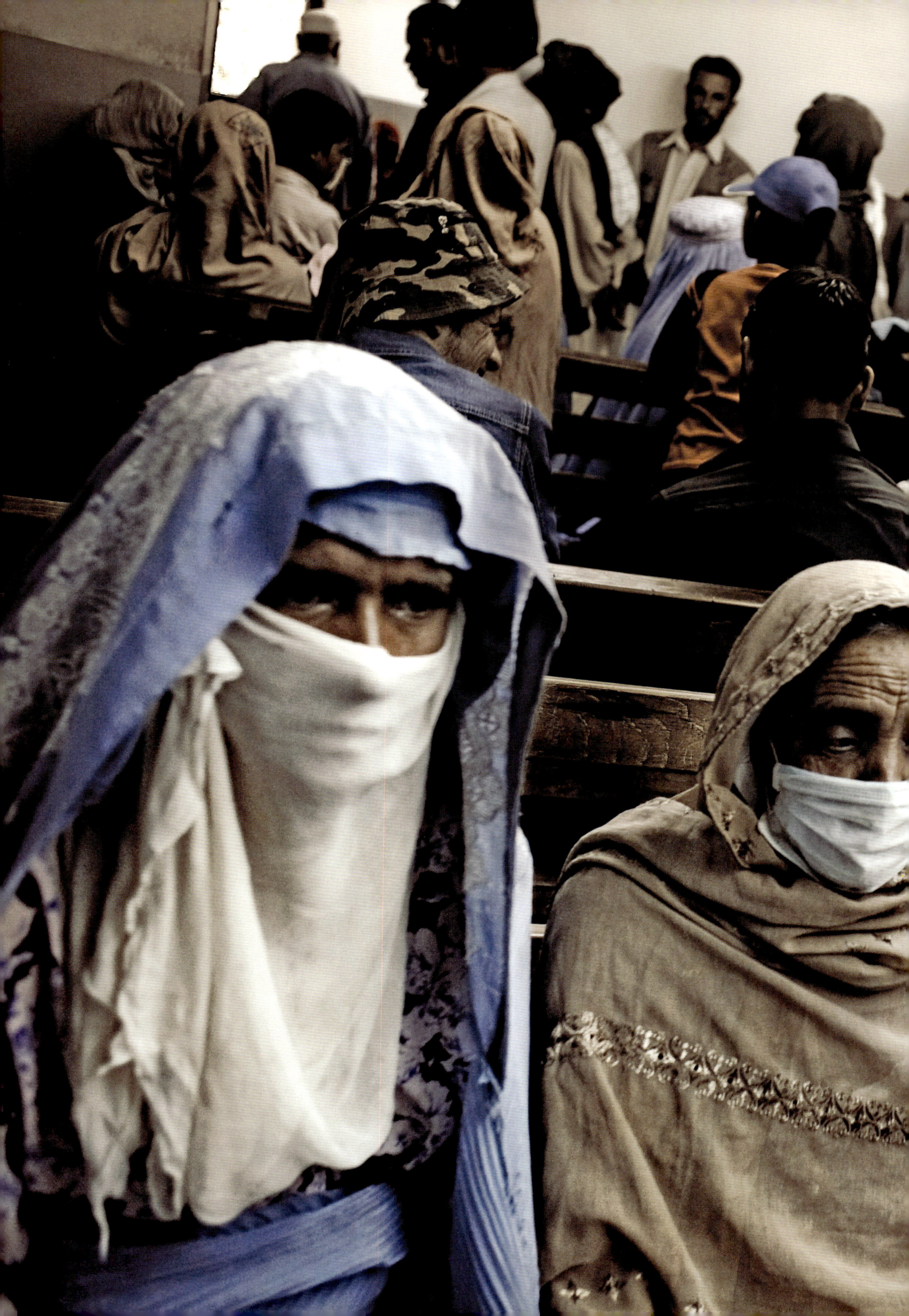

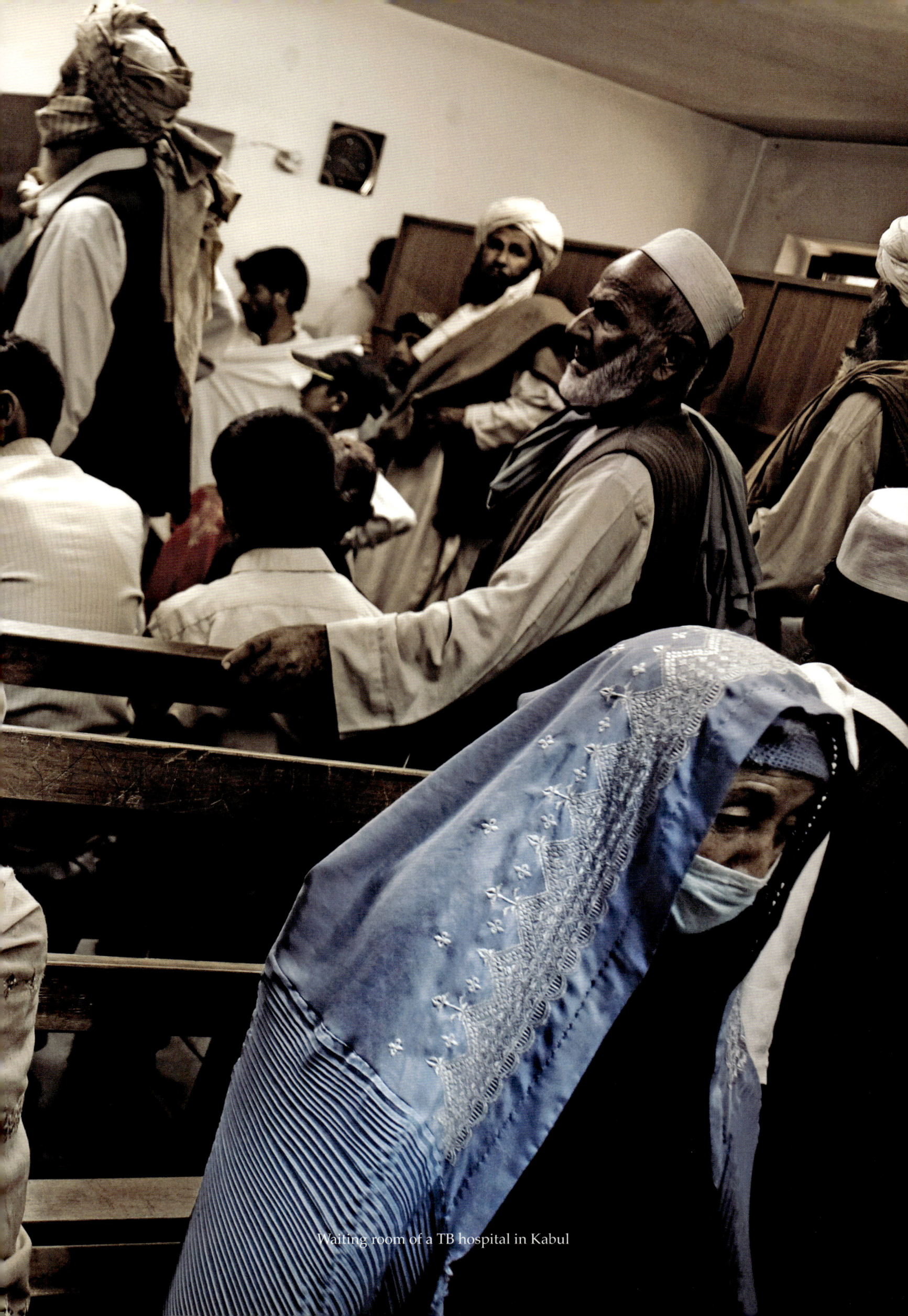
Waiting room of a TB hospital in Kabul

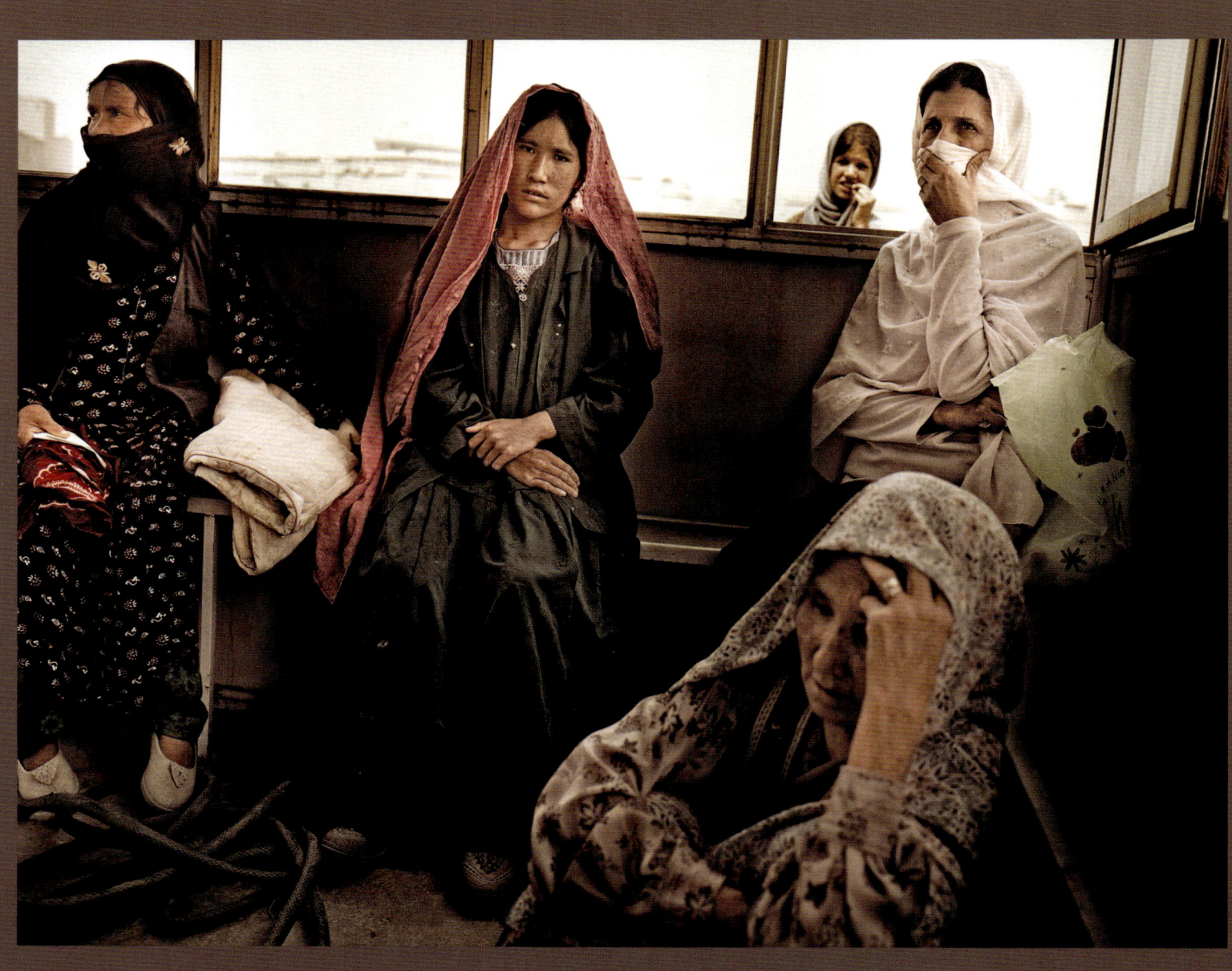

Sakina (centre) is 20 years old and has been receiving DOTS at the
National TB Hospital in Kabul for two months but is still not feeling well

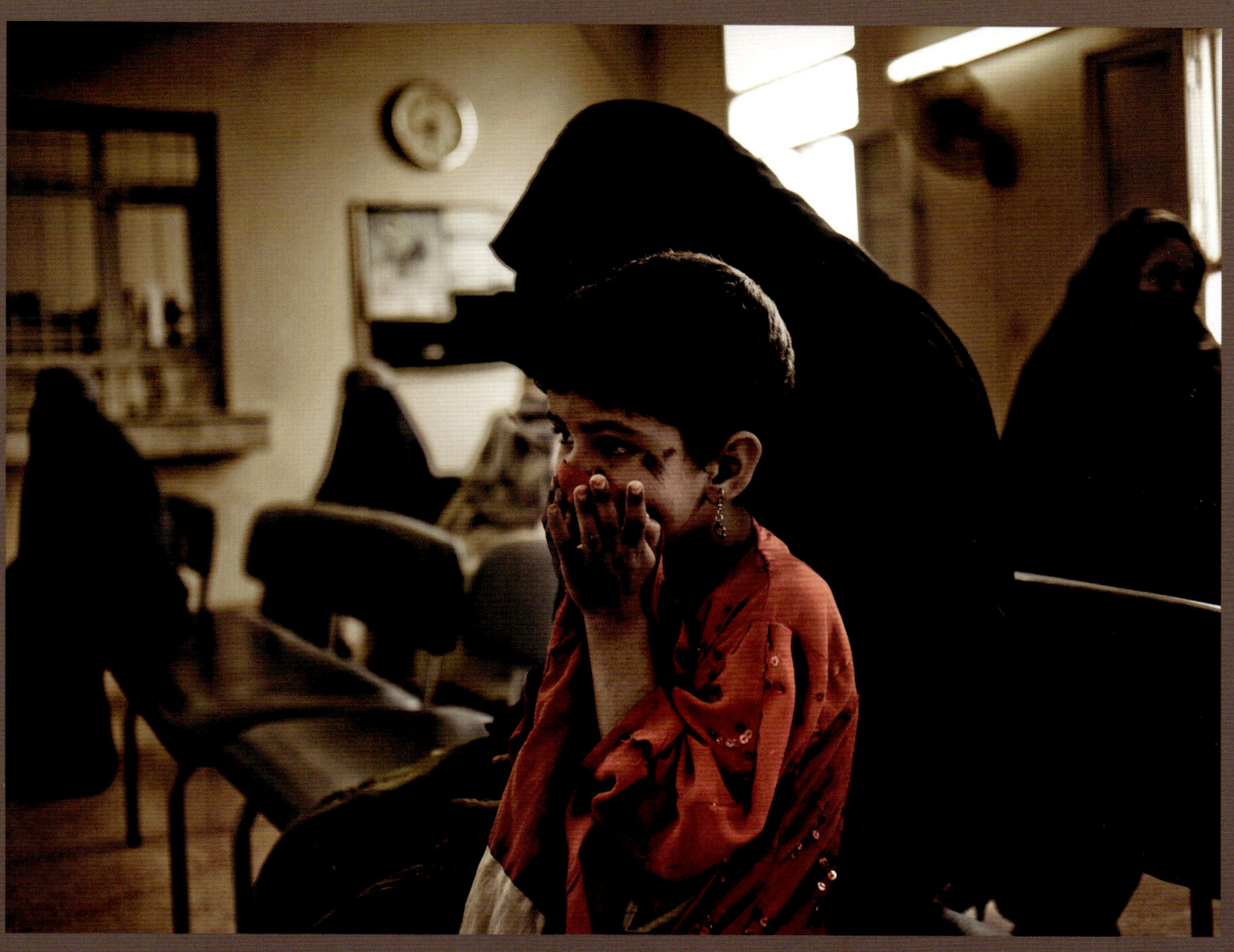

Fatima, 9 years old, waits with her mother for the results to confirm her diagnosis

Illness keeps you locked up... proper medication will break down the door

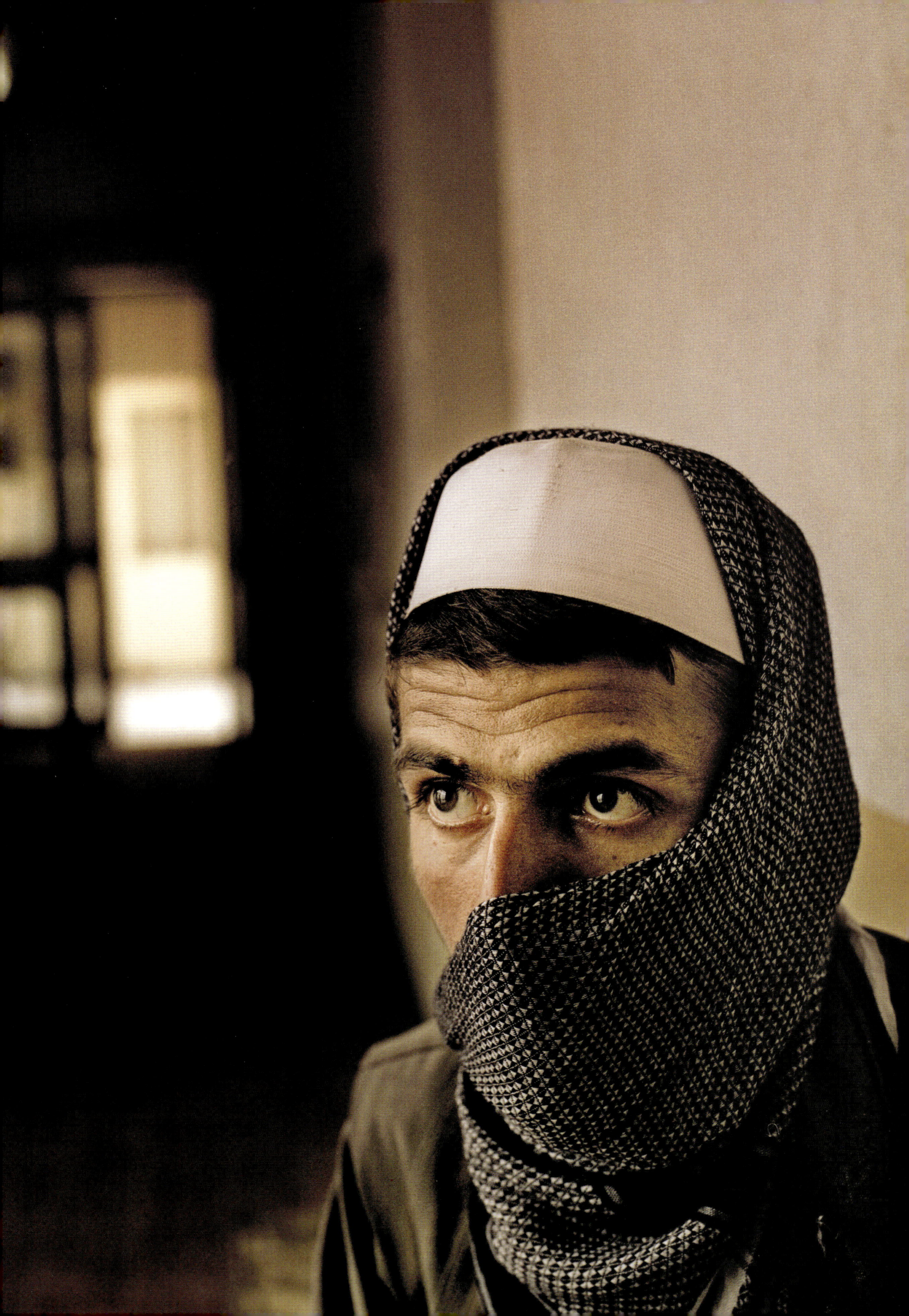

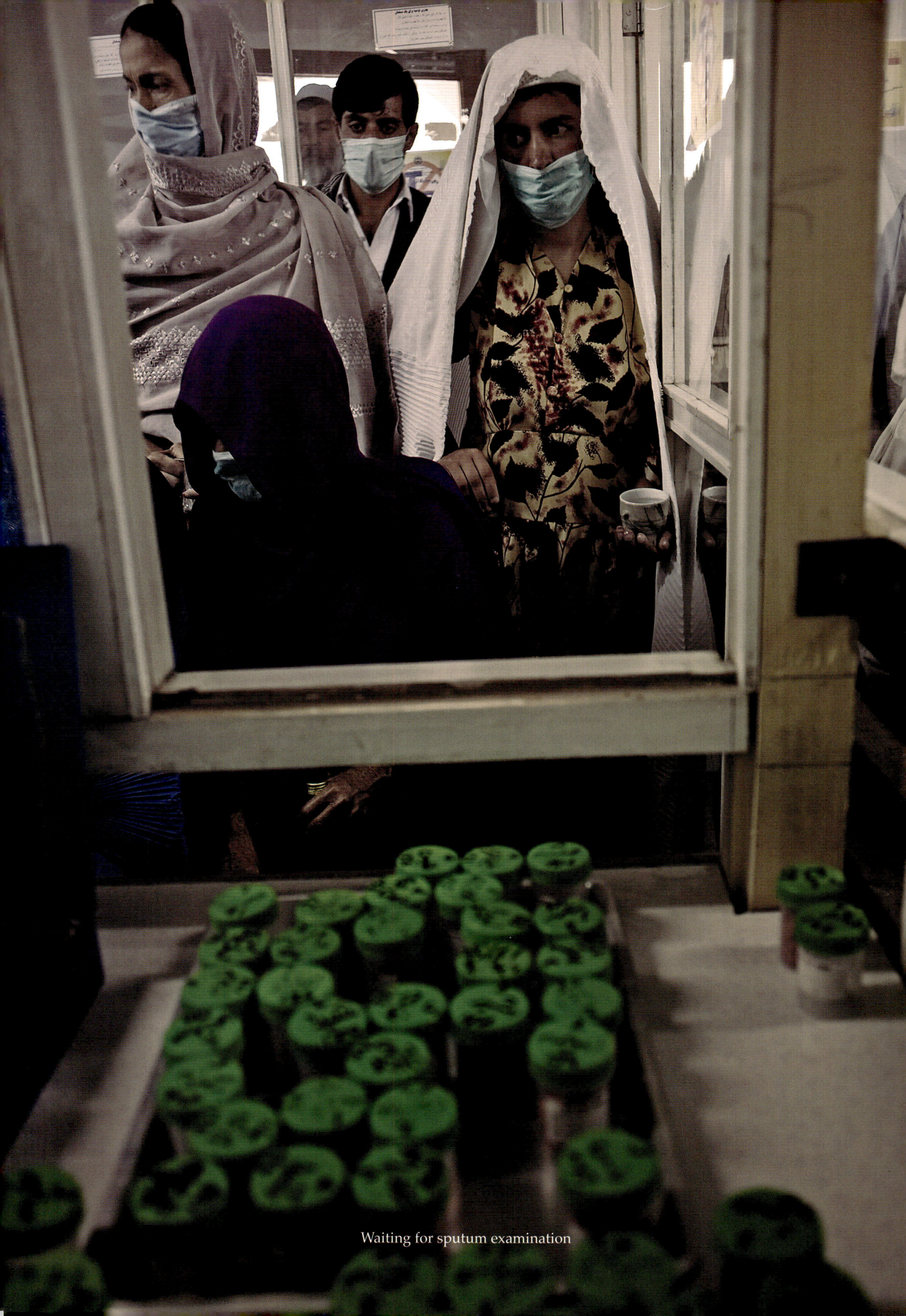
Waiting for sputum examination

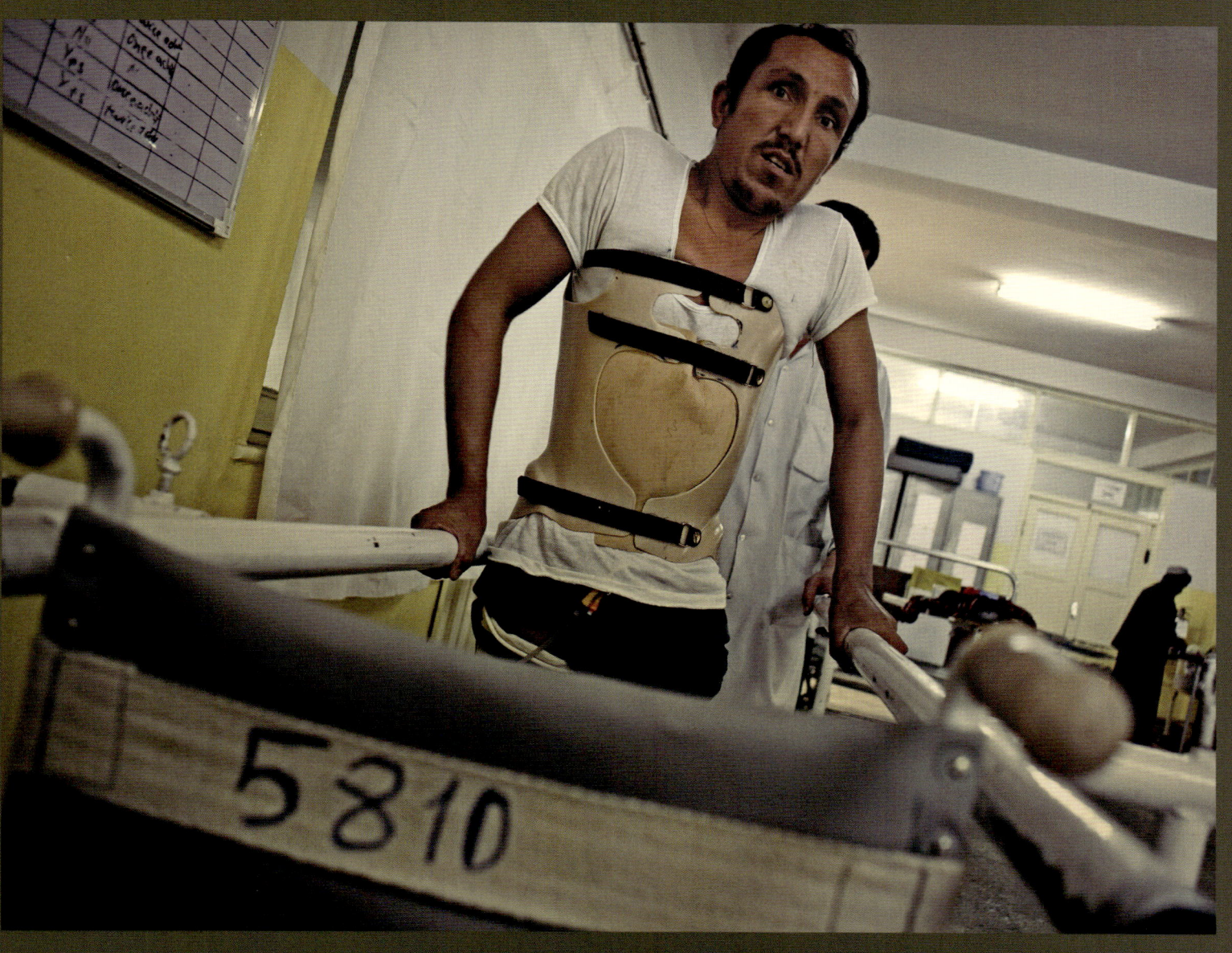

Omar undergoes his physiotherapy

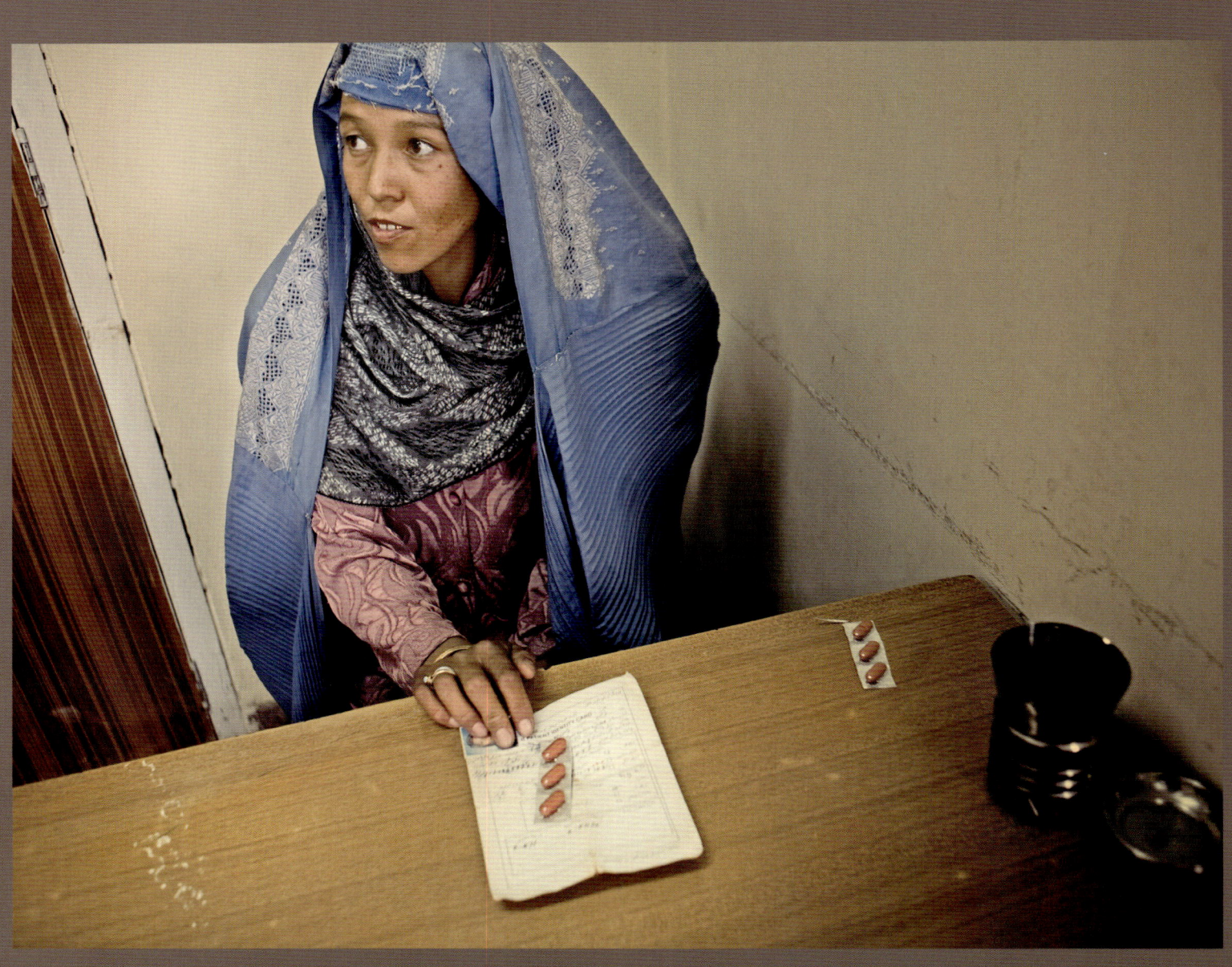

Supervised medication is the key to curing TB...

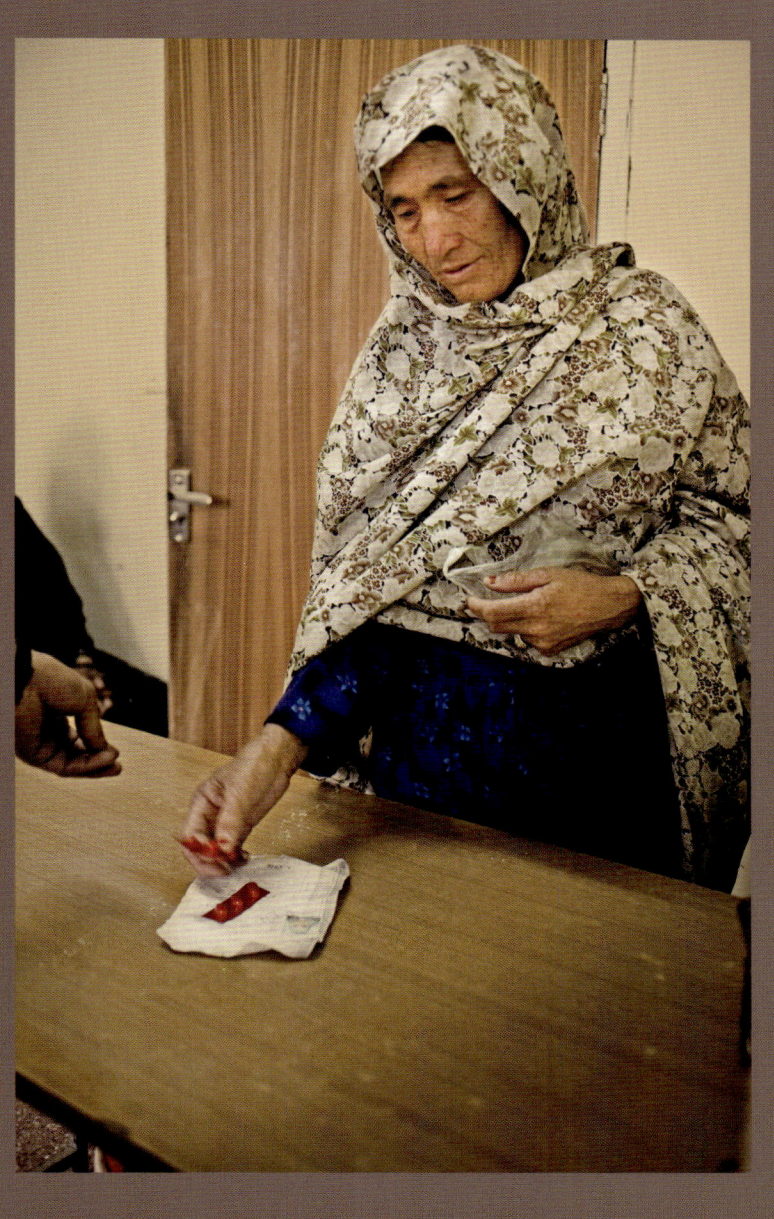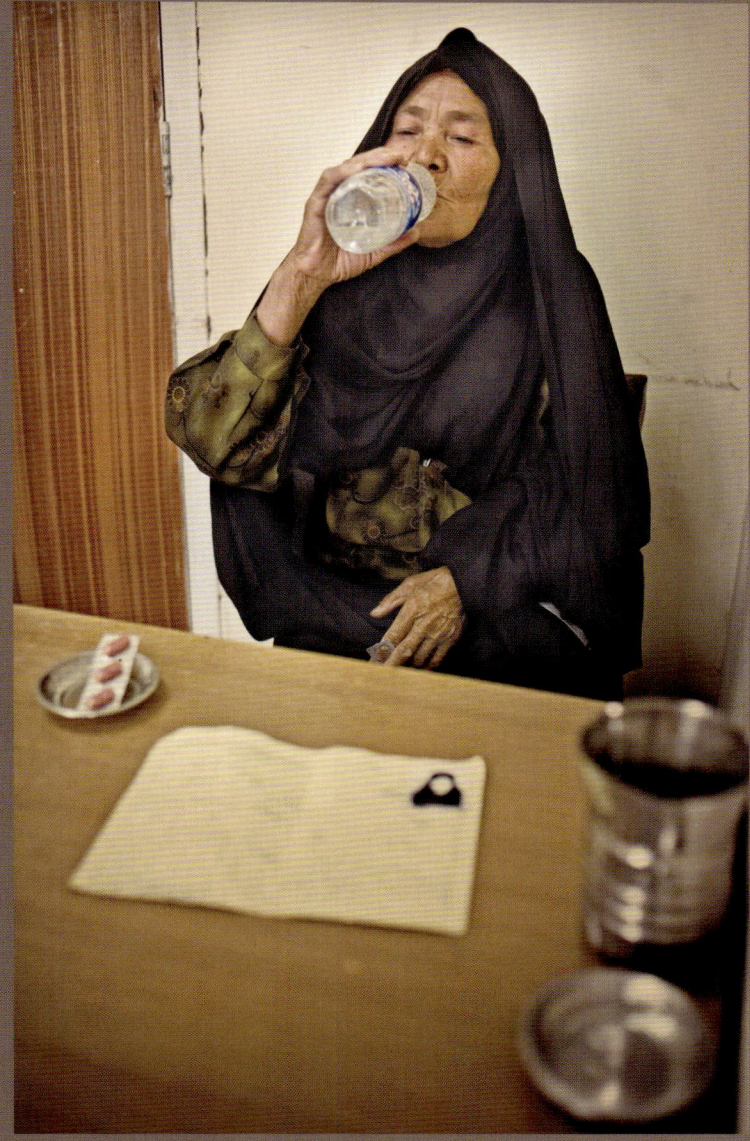

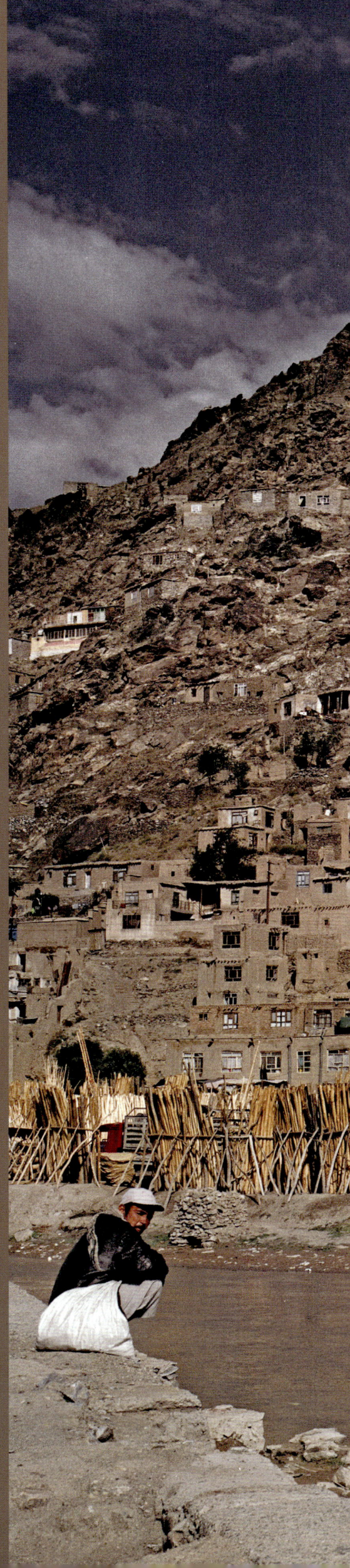

Behind every door dwells an unheard soul, gasping for air,
reaching out for help

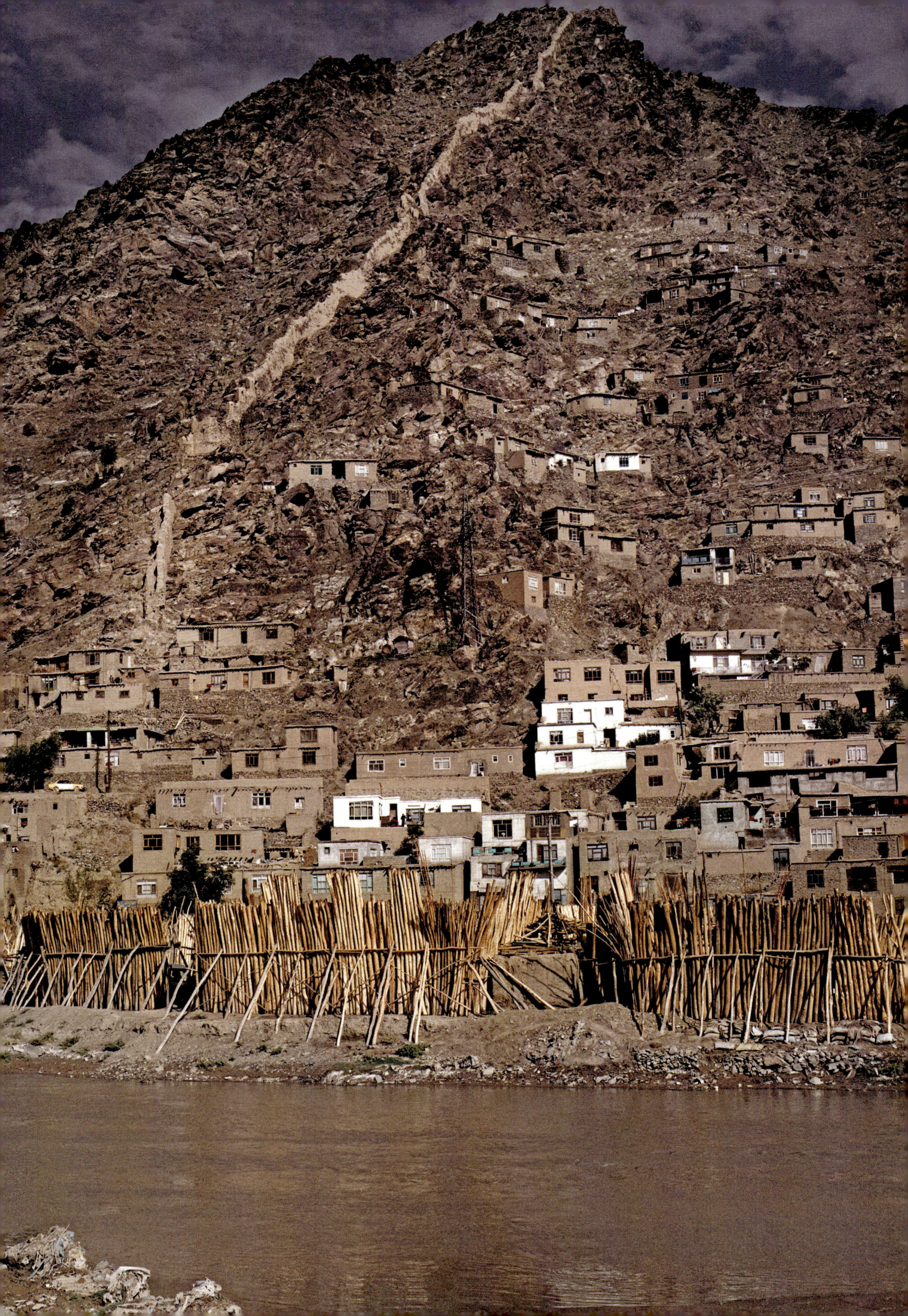

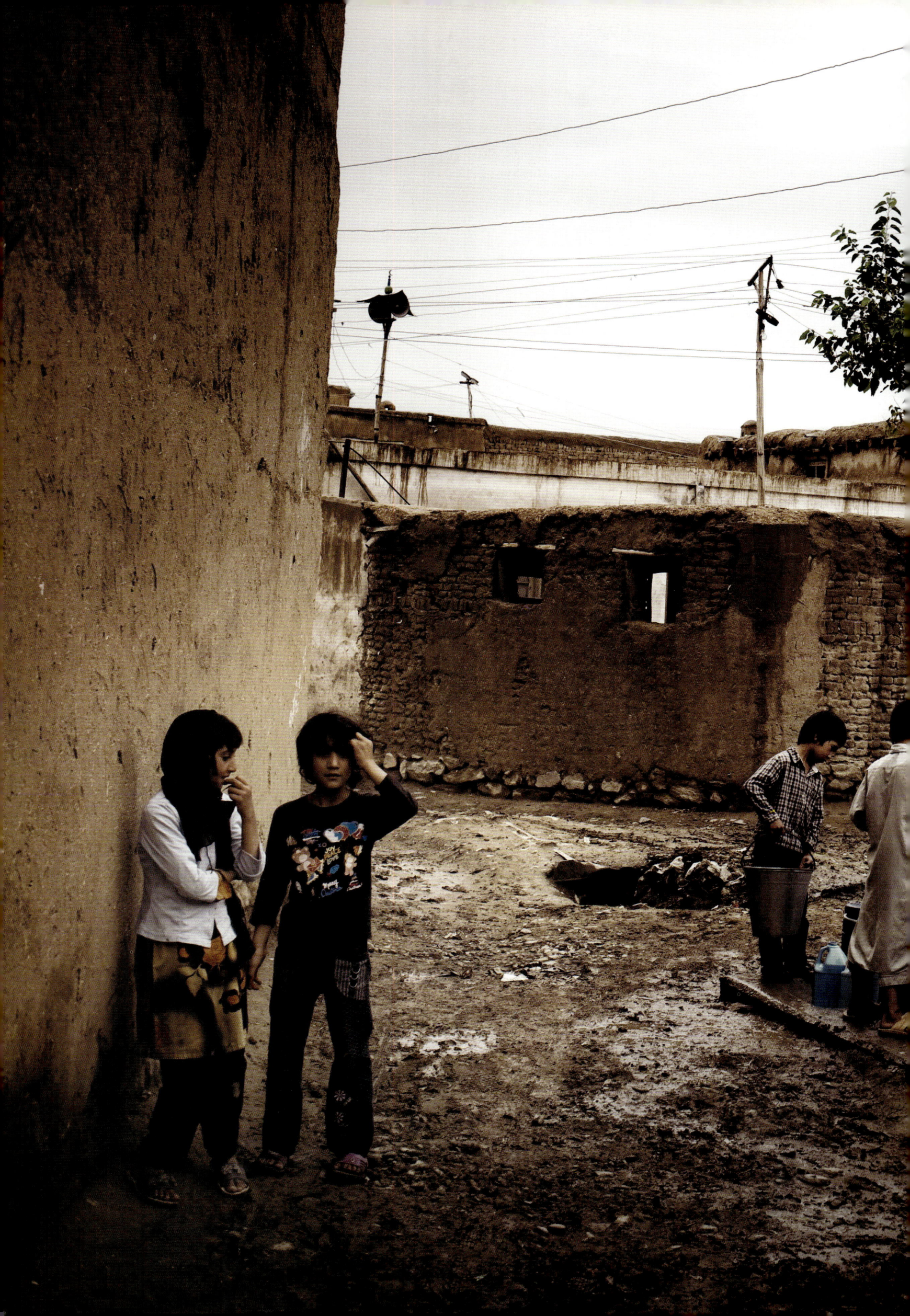

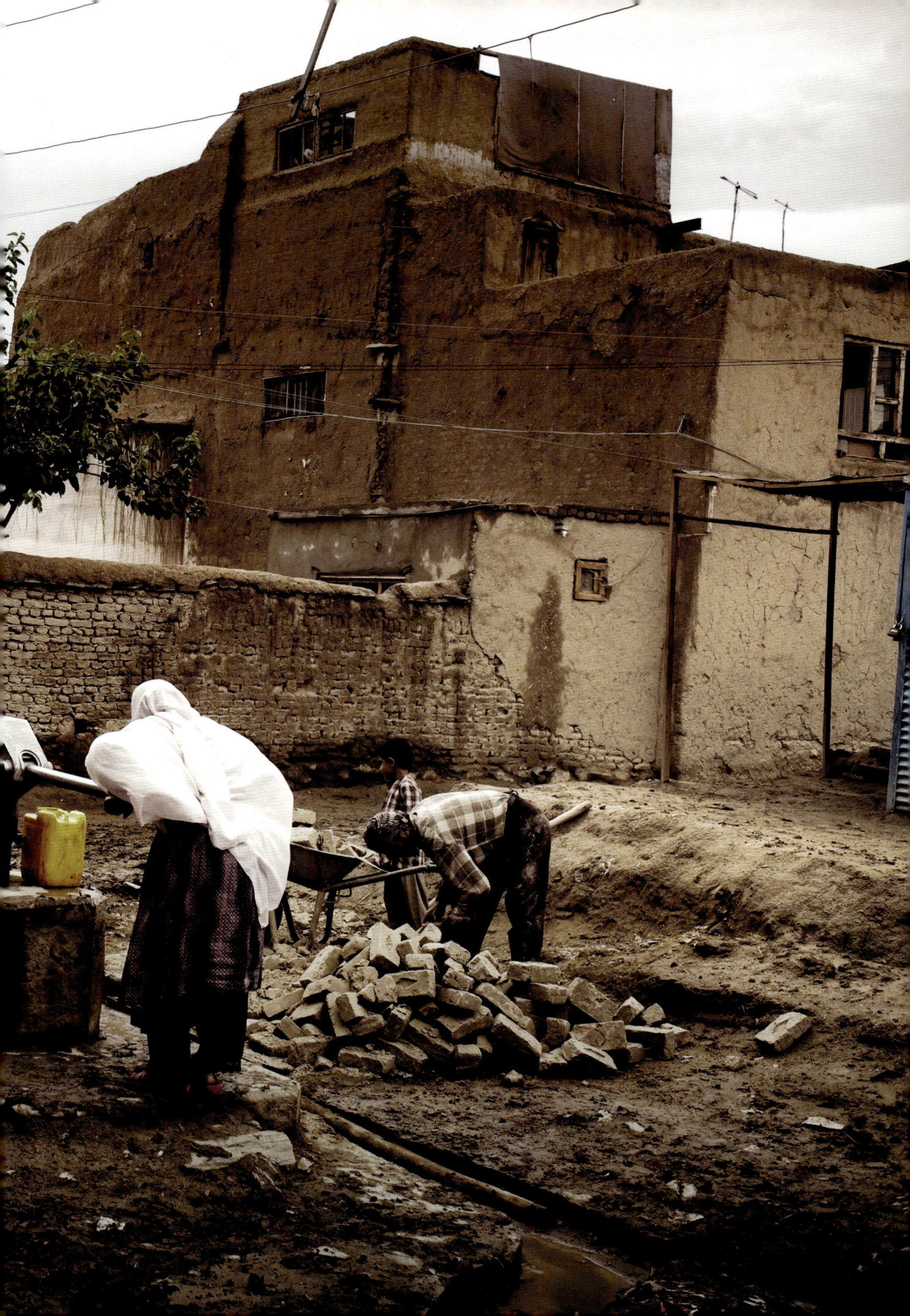

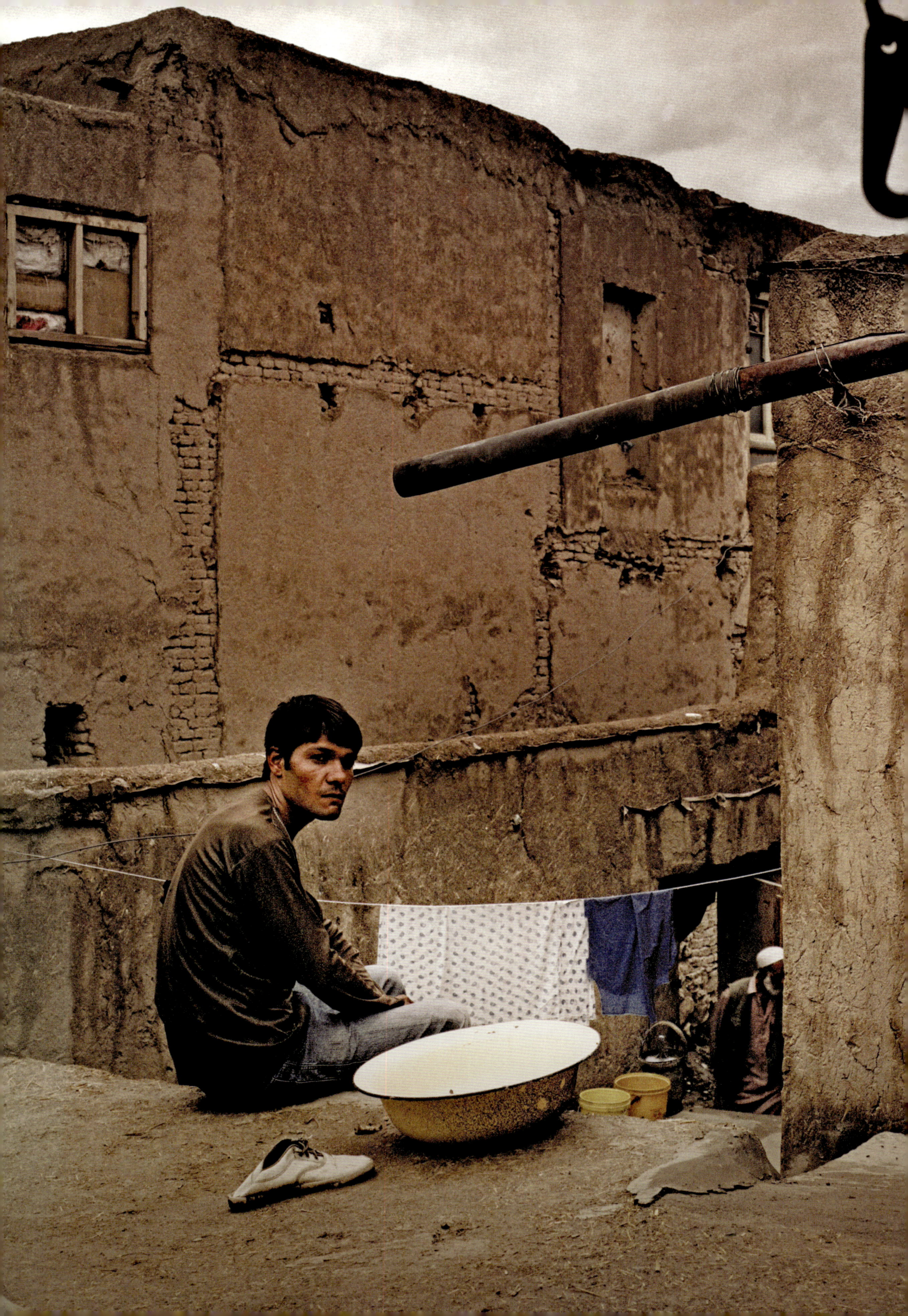

Ramatullah, a 25-year old bus conductor, has drug-resistant TB but must keep working to support his family

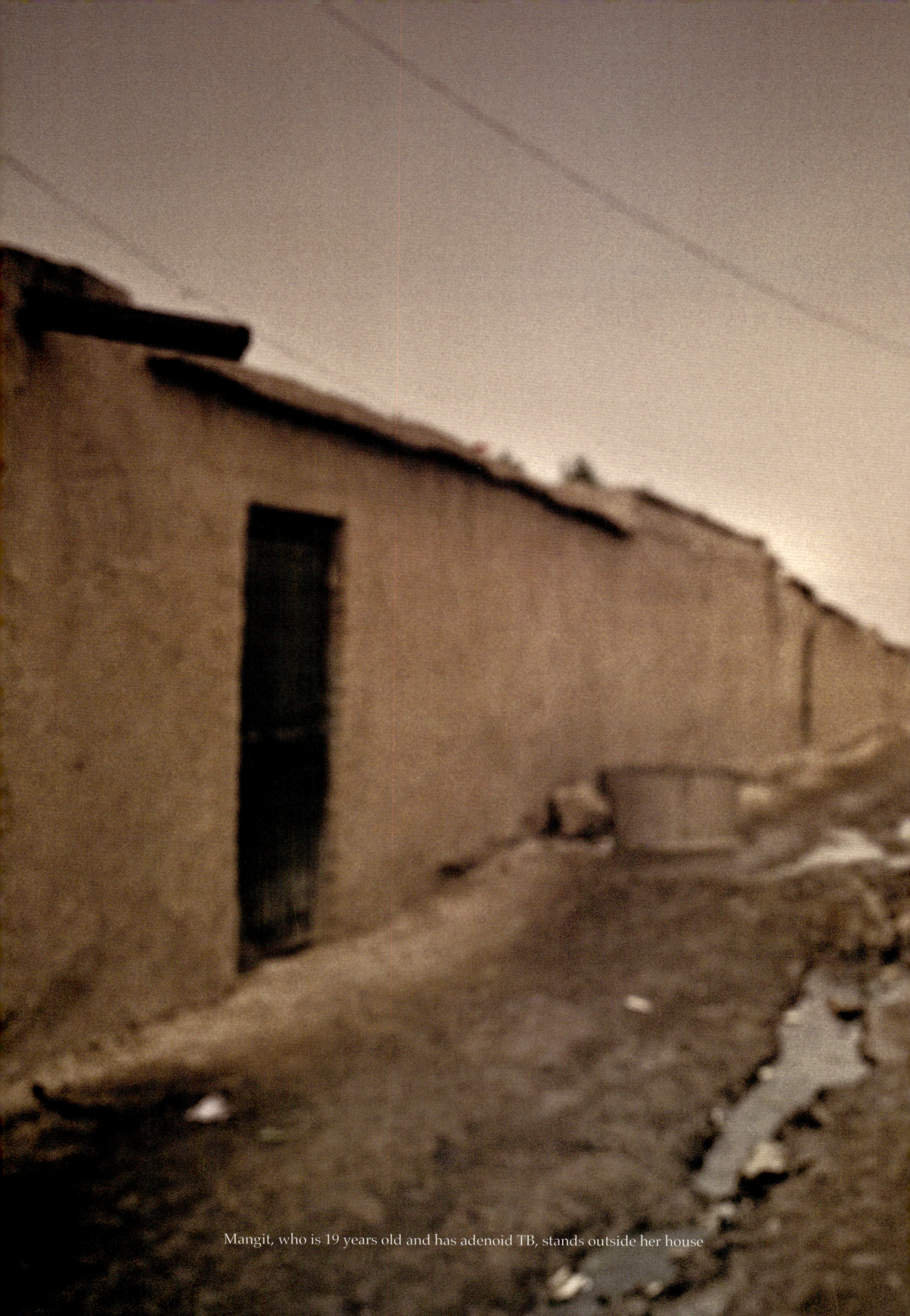

Mangit, who is 19 years old and has adenoid TB, stands outside her house

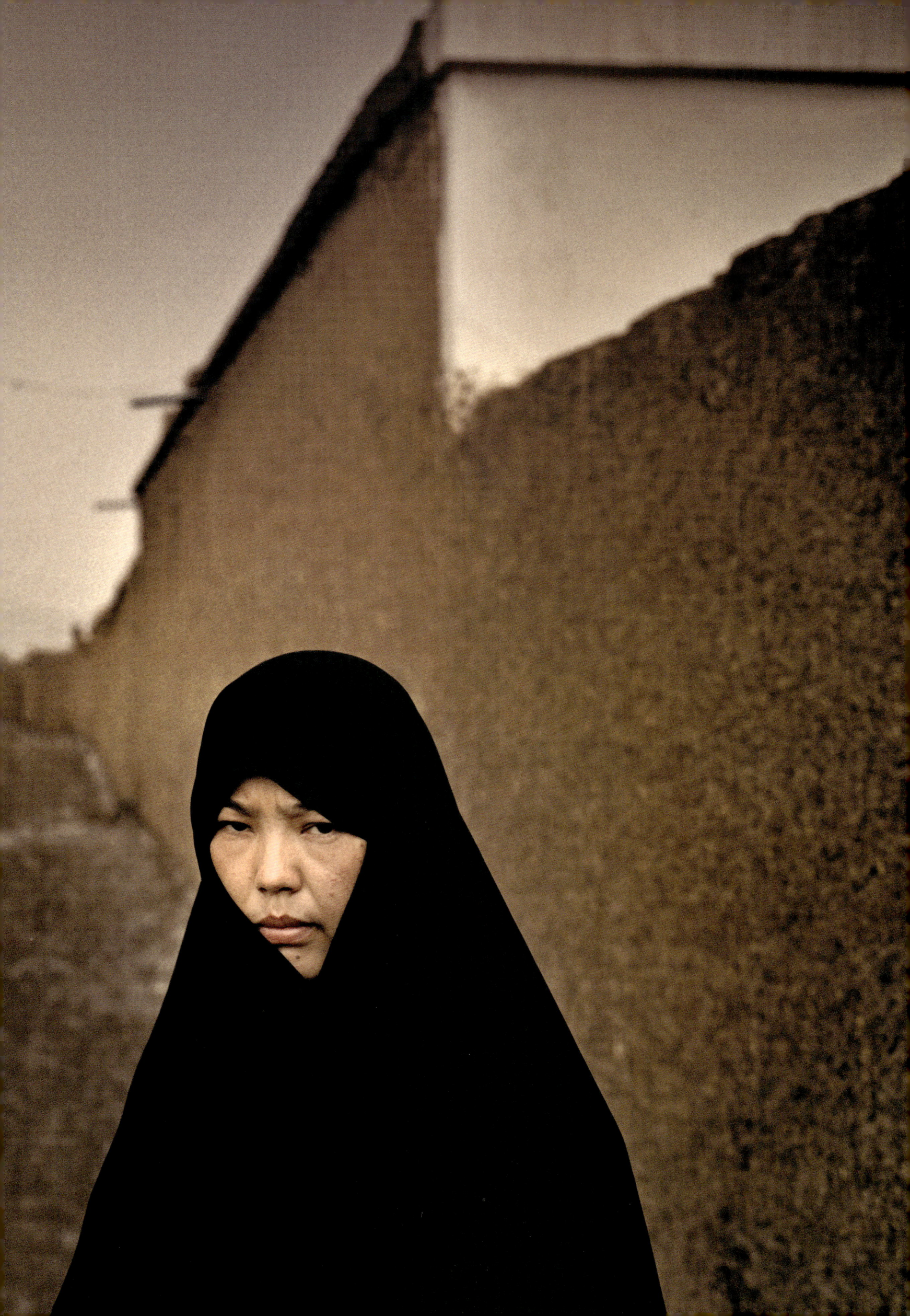

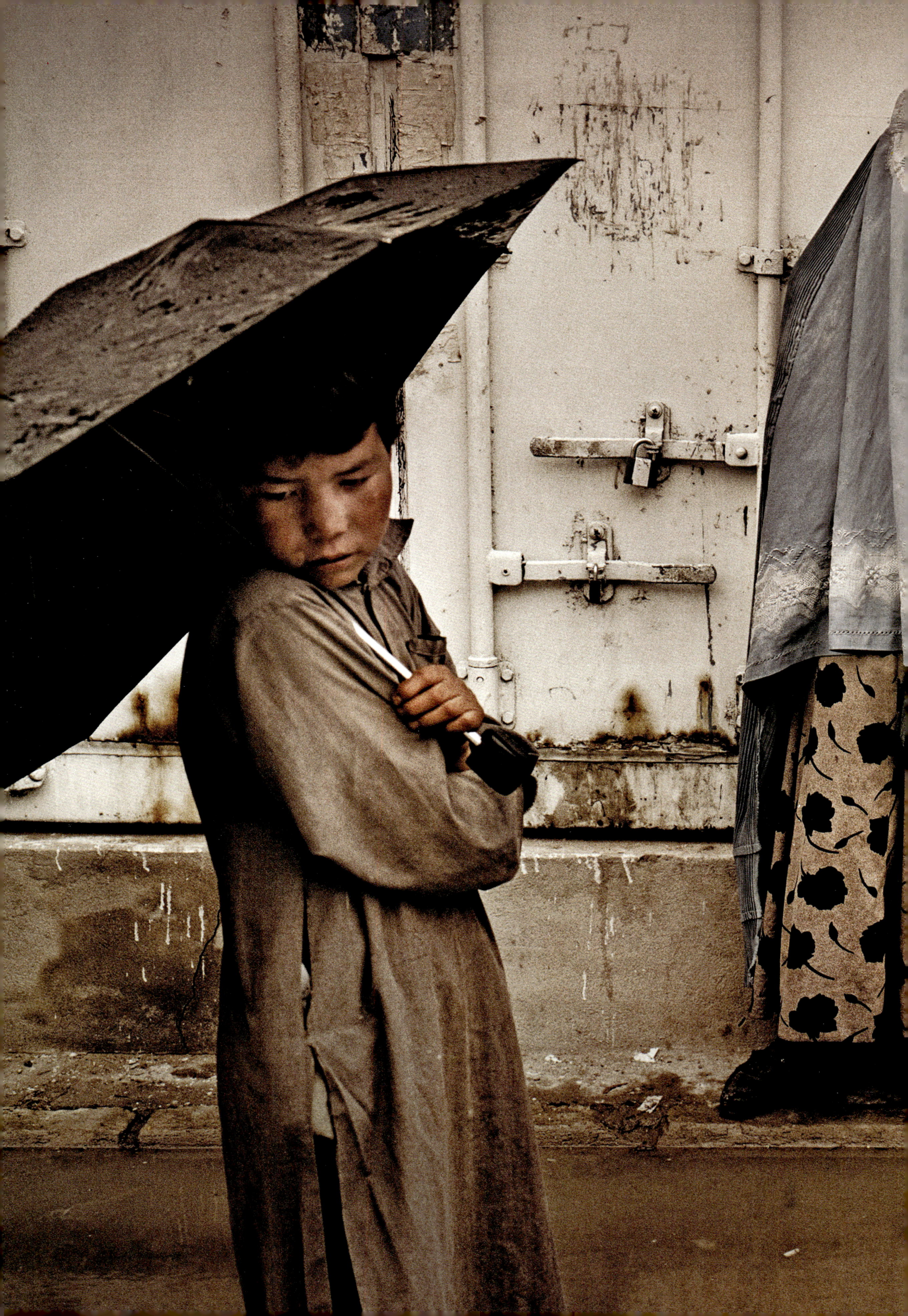

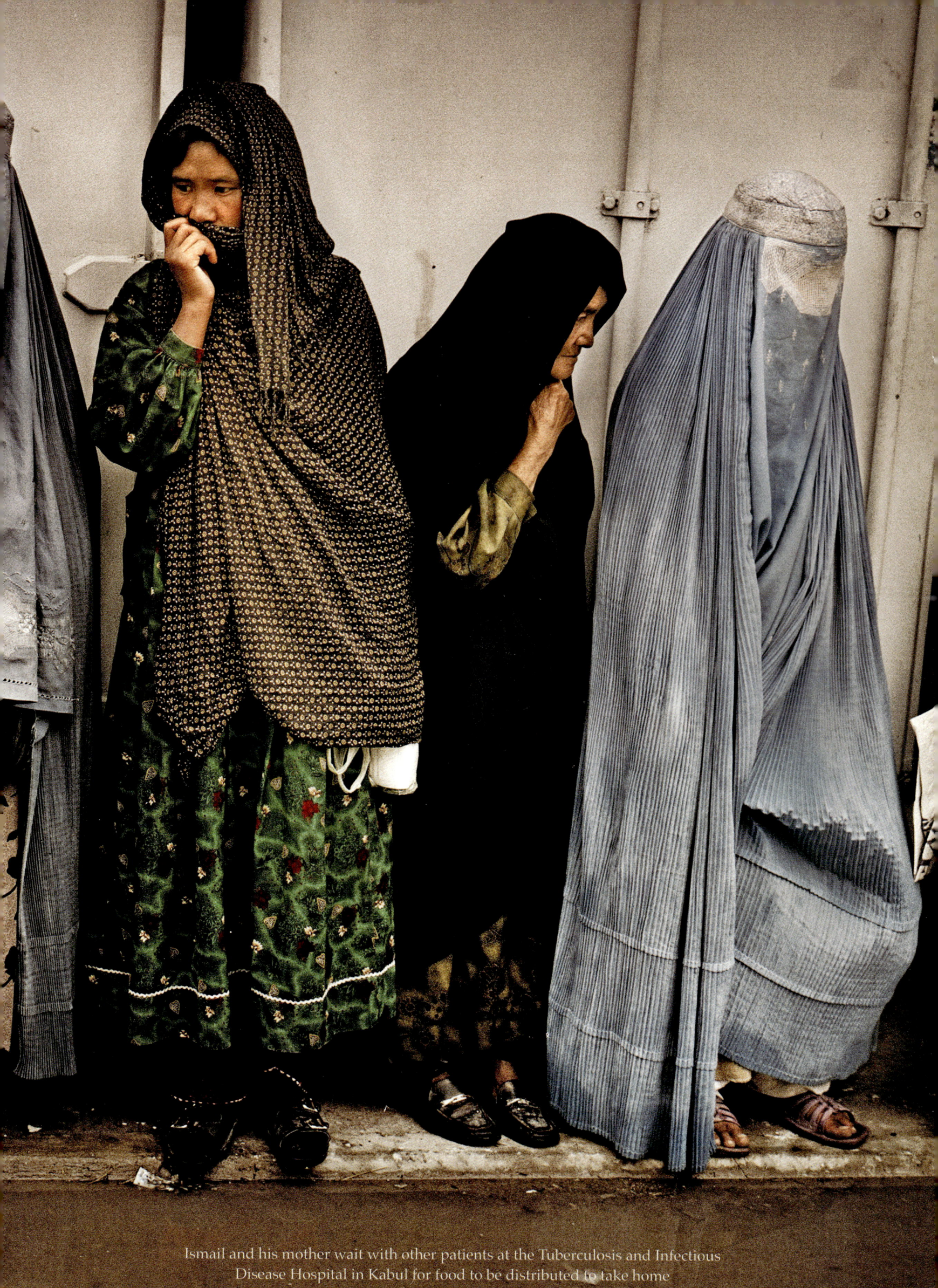
Ismail and his mother wait with other patients at the Tuberculosis and Infectious Disease Hospital in Kabul for food to be distributed to take home

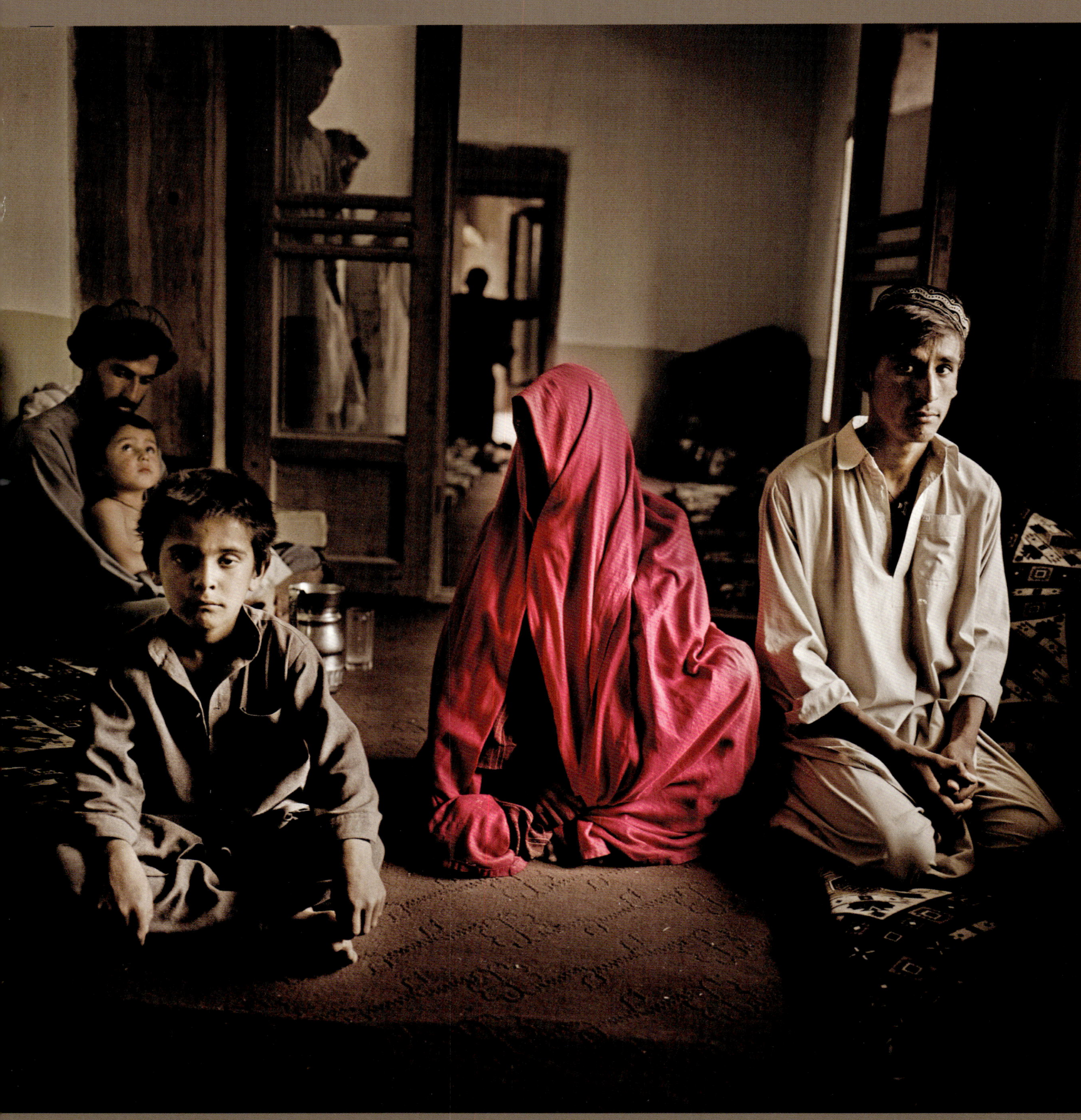
At home in Kabul, Lakten and her two grandsons all have TB